DEMENTIA

A Doctor's Practical Guide to Prevention & Early detection

Dr Prabhat Das

MD, PhD, FACP

Better Health with Dr Das Series

Hardcover ISBN: 978-1-971672-70-0

Paperback ISBN: 978-1-971672-69-4

eBook ISBN: 978-1-971672-68-7

Printed in the United States of America

Disclaimer

This book is intended solely for educational and informational purposes. It is not meant to replace personal medical advice, diagnosis, or treatment.

Although I am a licensed physician, reading this book does not establish a doctor-patient relationship. Each individual's health condition, medical history, and risk factors are unique. Any medical decision should be made in partnership with your own healthcare professional who understands your specific situation.

Medical science is continually advancing. New research and updated guidelines may lead to changes in recommendations over time.

TABLE OF CONTENTS:

About the Author

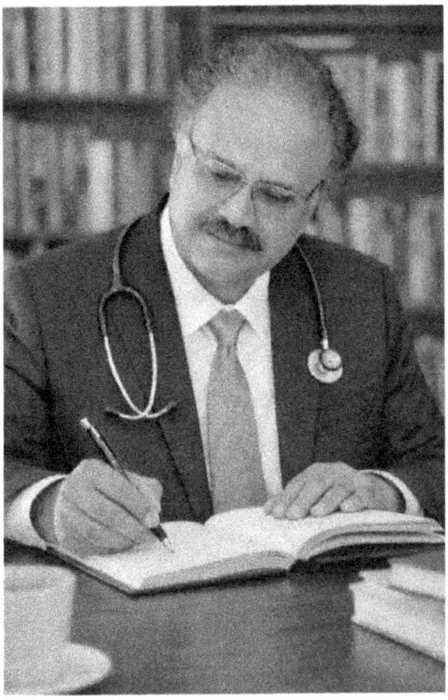

I am Dr Prabhat Das, MD, PhD, FACP. My journey in medicine began in India and, over the past thirty-five years, has continued in the United States, where I have had the privilege of caring for patients across a wide range of medical settings. I am trained in Internal Medicine, Pulmonary Diseases, and Critical Care. For me, medicine has never been just a profession. It has been a lifelong commitment shaped by learning, service, and a deep respect for the trust patients place in their physician.

Over the years, I have had the honor of caring for patients in many different situations. I have seen individuals in my office for routine concerns, treated urgent conditions in busy emergency rooms, managed serious illnesses in the hospital, and cared for critically ill patients in intensive care units. Each setting has taught me something valuable. Each patient has added to my understanding of what it truly means to care for another human being.

But one lesson has stood above all others. Medicine is not only about tests, diagnoses, or treatments. It is about people. It is about listening carefully, understanding fears that are often left unspoken, and guiding patients through uncertainty with clarity and compassion. Again and again, I have seen that what people want most is simple, trustworthy information. They want to understand what is happening in their bodies. They want to feel confident about the decisions they are making for their health and for their families.

These experiences have deeply shaped how I think about health, illness, prevention, and the human side of healing.

That is the reason behind the '**Better Health with Dr Das Series**'. Through these books, I hope to reach individuals I may never meet in person but who are searching for clear and reliable guidance. In today's world, health information is everywhere, yet much of it is confusing, overwhelming, and sometimes misleading. My goal is to cut through that noise and present important medical topics in a way that is simple, practical, and reassuring.

Every page of this series is guided by two foundations: reliable scientific knowledge and decades of real-world clinical experience. I want you, the reader, to feel informed, confident, and empowered. Not overwhelmed. Not confused. But clear about what you can do, step by step, to improve your health.

If even one reader feels less anxious, more informed, or better prepared to take control of their health after reading these books, then this work has served its purpose.

Helping people live healthier, longer, more confident and better-informed lives remains one of the greatest privileges of my life.

CHAPTER 1: When Memory Begins to Change

The Quiet Beginning That Families Often Miss

Dementia rarely begins with something dramatic.

There is no clear starting point. No single moment that tells you something serious has begun.

Instead, it begins quietly.

A name that does not come to mind.
A question repeated after a few minutes.
An item placed somewhere and never found again.

At first, these moments feel familiar. We all forget things. We smile, we reassure, and we move on.

"This is normal with age," we tell ourselves.

And many times, that is true.

But sometimes, there is a subtle difference.

The forgetfulness is not occasional anymore. It starts to repeat. It begins to interfere, quietly at first, with daily life.

That is the moment when we should not ignore it.

Not panic.
Not assume the worst.

But pause, observe, and take it seriously.

Normal Aging vs Dementia – A Crucial Difference

As we grow older, some degree of forgetfulness is expected.

You may forget where you kept your keys. You may struggle to recall a name. You may walk into a room and wonder why you came there.

In most cases, the memory returns.

This is normal aging.

Dementia is different.

The difference is not just memory. It is the **impact on daily life**.

In normal aging:

- You forget, but remember later
- You misplace things, but find them
- You remain independent
- Your judgment remains intact

In dementia:

- The memory does not return
- Questions are repeated frequently
- Familiar tasks become difficult
- Judgment may be impaired
- Daily functioning begins to decline

This distinction is very important.

Memory loss alone is not the issue.

Loss of independence is.

Why Families Often Wait Too Long

In real life, families often delay seeking help.

Not because they do not care.

But because:

- They hope things will improve
- They fear the diagnosis
- They are unsure if it is serious
- They do not want to upset the patient

Sometimes, there is quiet denial.

Sometimes, there is love behind the delay.

A spouse may feel, "I should not question him."
A child may feel, "Maybe I am overthinking."

But delay has a cost.

Early evaluation does not mean accepting a diagnosis immediately. It means understanding what is happening.

Some causes of memory problems are treatable.

Even when dementia is present, early stages allow:

- Better planning
- Safer decisions
- Patient involvement in future choices

That opportunity should not be missed.

Early Signs That Should Not Be Ignored

The earliest signs are often subtle.

But they are usually **progressive and repetitive**.

You may notice:

- Repeating the same questions
- Forgetting recent conversations
- Misplacing items frequently
- Difficulty managing bills or medications
- Trouble finding words
- Getting confused about dates or time
- Losing way in familiar places
- Changes in personality or behavior

Any one of these, once in a while, may not be serious.

But when they become a pattern, they deserve attention.

A Real-Life Reflection

I have seen this many times in my practice.

A person who was once very organized begins missing small details.

A careful planner starts forgetting appointments.

A confident driver becomes unsure on familiar roads.

At first, the family adjusts. They remind. They help. They compensate.

But slowly, the pattern becomes clearer.

It is not one mistake.

It is a change.

Recognizing that change is often the turning point.

The Emotional Side of Memory Changes

This stage is not only medical.

It is deeply emotional.

For the patient:

- There may be fear
- A sense of losing control
- Embarrassment in social situations

Many patients are aware, at least in the beginning, that something is not right.

For the family:

- Concern slowly builds
- Frustration may appear
- Guilt often follows

It is important to remember:

This is not intentional behavior.

The brain is beginning to change.

Understanding this replaces frustration with patience.

Why Early Evaluation Matters

Early evaluation is one of the most important steps.

It helps answer critical questions:

- Is this normal aging?
- Is this mild cognitive impairment?

- Is this dementia?
- Is there a reversible cause?

Many conditions can mimic dementia, including:

- Medication side effects
- Depression
- Sleep disorders
- Vitamin deficiencies
- Thyroid problems

Identifying these can make a real difference.

Even when dementia is diagnosed, early recognition allows:

- Better safety planning
- Medication review
- Legal and financial planning
- Emotional preparation

Early clarity reduces future crises.

Doctor's Pearl

When memory changes are repeated, progressive, and affecting daily life, do not ignore them. Early evaluation is a wise and necessary step.

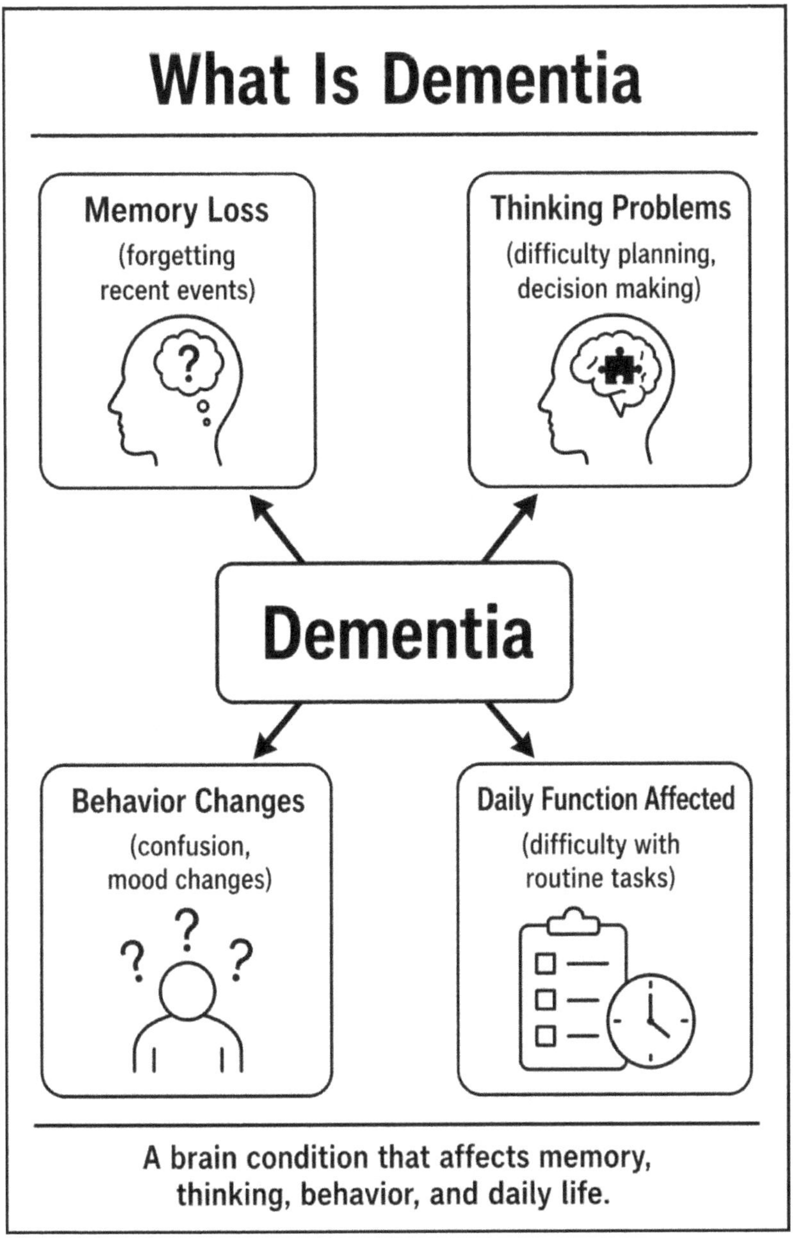
What Is Dementia
Memory Loss
(forgetting recent events)
?
Thinking Problems
(difficulty planning, decision making)
Dementia
Behavior Changes
(confusion, mood changes)
? ? ?
Daily Function Affected
(difficulty with routine tasks)
A brain condition that affects memory, thinking, behavior, and daily life.

Myth vs Fact

Myth: Memory loss is a normal part of aging.
Fact: Mild forgetfulness can occur, but memory loss that interferes with daily life is not normal and should be evaluated.

Common Mistakes to Avoid

- Ignoring repeated symptoms
- Blaming everything on aging
- Waiting for a crisis before acting
- Arguing with the patient
- Avoiding medical consultation due to fear

Red Flag Warnings

- Repeating the same questions frequently
- Getting lost in familiar places
- Difficulty managing medications or finances
- Noticeable personality change
- Unsafe decisions or behavior
- Rapid worsening over weeks or months

Chapter Summary

Memory changes often begin quietly and are easy to overlook.

Normal aging causes mild forgetfulness, but dementia affects daily life, judgment, and independence.
Early signs are subtle but progressive.
Recognizing patterns early allows timely evaluation and better planning.

Action Plan

- Observe changes over time
- Keep simple notes of repeated issues
- Discuss concerns with family members
- Seek medical evaluation if symptoms persist
- Bring a family member to the doctor visit
- Do not delay due to fear or uncertainty

Transition to Next Chapter

Now that we understand how memory changes begin and why early attention matters, the next step is to clearly understand what dementia really is, how it affects the brain, and why these changes occur.

CHAPTER 2: What Dementia Really Means

A Word That Creates Fear, and Why It Should Not

In my practice, I have seen how a single word can change the entire atmosphere in a room.

The moment the word "dementia" is mentioned, there is often silence. Faces become serious. Questions remain unspoken.

For many people, dementia means loss. Loss of memory, independence, identity, and connection.

That fear is understandable.

But before we allow fear to take over, we must understand one important truth.

Dementia is not one single disease.

It is a medical condition with different causes, different patterns, and different outcomes.

When we understand it clearly, we replace fear with clarity.

And clarity changes everything.

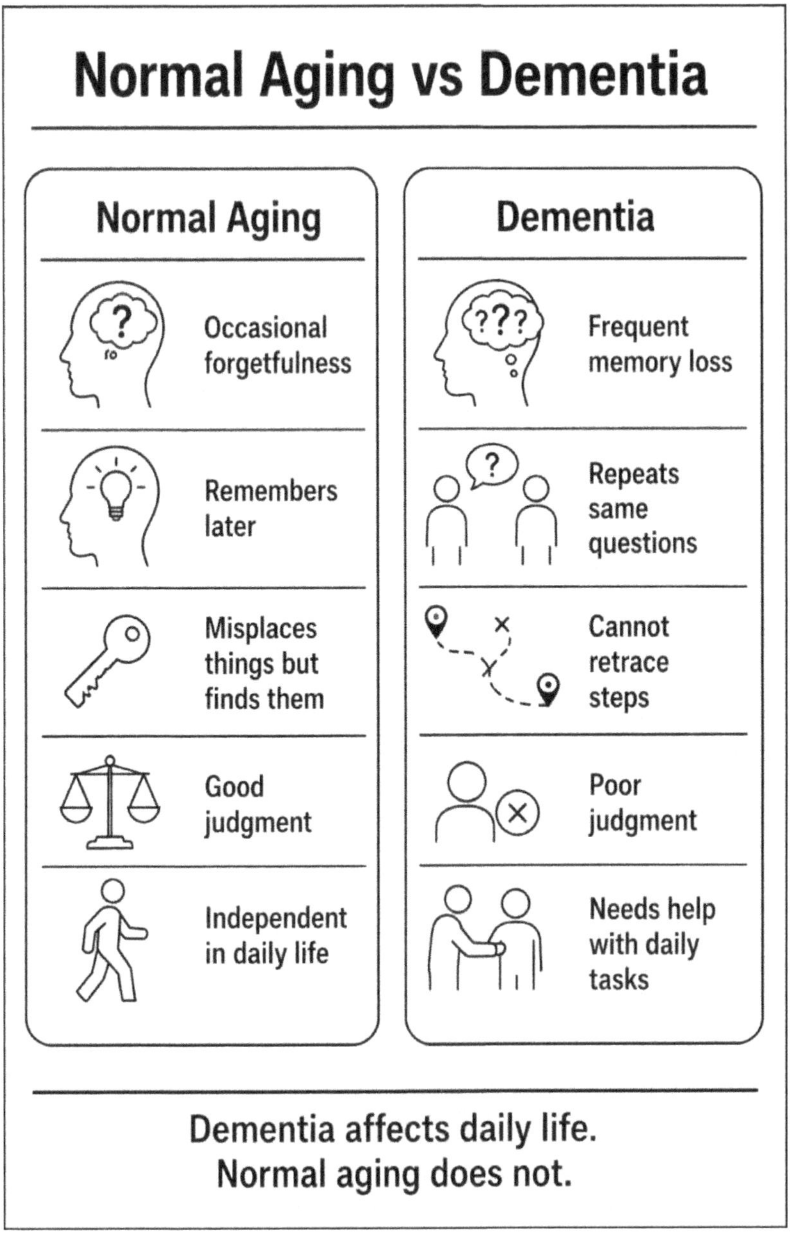
Normal Aging vs Dementia
Normal Aging
Occasional forgetfulness
Remembers later
Misplaces things but finds them
Good judgment
Independent in daily life
Dementia
Frequent memory loss
Repeats same questions
Cannot retrace steps
Poor judgment
Needs help with daily tasks
Dementia affects daily life.
Normal aging does not.

Dementia Is a Syndrome, Not a Single Disease

Dementia is what we call a **syndrome**.

This means a group of symptoms that occur together.

These symptoms affect:

- Memory
- Thinking
- Judgment
- Language
- Behavior
- Ability to perform daily activities

Several different diseases can cause these symptoms.

The most common cause is Alzheimer's disease, but there are many others.

This distinction is important.

Because understanding the cause helps us understand:

- What to expect
- How the condition may progress
- How best to manage it

It Is Not Just About Memory

One of the biggest misconceptions is that dementia is only a memory problem.

Memory loss is often the first symptom, but it is not the whole story.

Dementia affects multiple areas of brain function.

A person may begin to have difficulty with:

- Planning and organizing
- Following conversations
- Making decisions
- Managing finances
- Performing familiar tasks

Over time, even simple daily activities may become challenging.

This is what separates dementia from normal forgetfulness.

How Dementia Affects the Brain

To understand dementia, it helps to think of the brain as a highly organized system.

Different areas of the brain have different roles:

- The hippocampus helps form new memories
- The frontal lobes control judgment, planning, and behavior

- The temporal lobes are involved in language and understanding
- The parietal lobes help with spatial awareness

In dementia, these areas are gradually damaged.

This damage may occur due to:

- Abnormal protein accumulation
- Reduced blood supply
- Degeneration of brain cells

As more brain cells are affected, symptoms become more noticeable.

The process is usually slow, but it is progressive.

Different Causes, Similar Effects

There are several types of dementia, including:

- Alzheimer-type dementia
- Vascular dementia
- Lewy body dementia
- Frontotemporal dementia
- Mixed dementia

Each type has its own pattern.

Some begin with memory loss.
Others begin with behavior changes or movement problems.

But all of them affect the brain's ability to function.

This is why proper diagnosis matters.

Dementia, Delirium, and Depression – A Critical Distinction

In medical practice, one of the most important tasks is to distinguish dementia from other conditions that can look similar.

Dementia

- Gradual onset
- Slowly progressive
- Persistent symptoms

Delirium

- Sudden onset
- Fluctuating course
- Often caused by infection, medications, or illness
- Requires urgent attention

Depression

- May cause poor concentration and memory complaints
- Associated with low mood and lack of interest
- Often improves with treatment

Confusing these conditions can lead to serious mistakes.

Recognizing the difference is essential for proper care.

Why Daily Life Is Affected So Deeply

As dementia progresses, the brain loses its ability to manage complex tasks.

Activities that once felt automatic now require effort.

Tasks such as:

- Cooking
- Driving
- Managing medications
- Handling finances

may become difficult or unsafe.

This is not due to lack of effort.

It is due to real changes in brain function.

Understanding this helps families respond with patience instead of frustration.

The Human Side of Dementia

Beyond the medical explanation, dementia is deeply personal.

It affects identity.

A person who was once confident and independent may become uncertain or withdrawn.

Families often say, "He is not the same person anymore."

But it is important to remember something very important.

The person is still there.

They may struggle with memory and communication, but they still experience:

- Emotions
- Comfort and discomfort
- Connection with others

Care must always preserve these human elements.

A Real-Life Reflection

I once cared for a patient who had been a respected teacher.

In the early stages, he would pause in the middle of a sentence, searching for words.

He once said quietly, “I know what I want to say, but it is not coming.”

That moment stayed with me.

It reminded me that in early dementia, patients often understand more than we realize.

They need support, not correction.

Patience, not pressure.

Doctor’s Pearl

Dementia is not just memory loss. It affects thinking, behavior, and independence. When we understand this, we respond with empathy instead of frustration.

Myth vs Fact

Myth: Dementia and Alzheimer’s disease are the same.
Fact: Alzheimer’s disease is one cause of dementia. Several other conditions can also lead to dementia.

Common Mistakes to Avoid

- Assuming all dementia is the same
- Ignoring sudden confusion, which may be delirium

- Dismissing depression as normal aging
- Expecting the patient to function as before

Red Flag Warnings

- Sudden onset confusion
- Rapid decline over a short period
- New hallucinations or unusual behavior
- Difficulty performing routine daily tasks

Chapter Summary

Dementia is a syndrome caused by different diseases affecting the brain.
It involves memory, thinking, behavior, and daily functioning.
It is different from normal aging, delirium, and depression.
Understanding dementia clearly helps reduce fear and improves care.

Action Plan

- Learn the difference between normal aging and dementia
- Observe changes beyond memory
- Seek medical evaluation for sudden or unusual symptoms

- Avoid assumptions without proper diagnosis
- Support the patient with patience and understanding

Transition to Next Chapter

Now that we understand what dementia truly means, the next step is to recognize the early warning signs in daily life, so that no important signal is missed and timely action can be taken.

CHAPTER 3: Early Warning Signs Families Should Not Ignore

When Small Changes Begin to Tell a Story

In the early phase of dementia, nothing appears dramatic.

There is no clear moment that tells you something serious has begun.

Instead, there are small changes. Scattered. Subtle. Easy to overlook.

A repeated question.
A forgotten conversation.
A misplaced item that cannot be found.

Each of these, by itself, may seem harmless.

But over time, these small changes begin to form a pattern.

And that pattern is what matters.

In my experience, families often say later, “We noticed these things earlier, but we did not realize what they meant.”

This chapter is meant to help you recognize those early signals clearly, without confusion or fear.

Memory Changes That Go Beyond Normal Aging

We all forget things occasionally.

But in early dementia, memory problems behave differently.

You may notice:

- Repeating the same question within a short time
- Forgetting recent conversations completely
- Misplacing items and being unable to find them
- Increasing reliance on reminders

One important clue is this:

The person may not realize they are repeating themselves.

This is often noticed by family members first.

Problems with Thinking and Judgment

Dementia affects thinking, not just memory.

Early changes may include:

- Difficulty planning or organizing
- Trouble following conversations
- Poor financial decisions
- Reduced problem-solving ability

A person who once handled finances carefully may begin making unusual errors.

This is not carelessness.

It reflects a change in brain function.

Getting Lost in Familiar Places

This is a very important warning sign.

A person may:

- Take a wrong turn on a familiar route
- Forget how to return home
- Become confused in well-known surroundings

Even if it happens once, it should not be ignored.

Safety becomes a concern early in such cases.

Changes in Language and Communication

Communication may gradually become difficult.

You may notice:

- Difficulty finding the right words
- Pausing frequently during conversation
- Losing track of what they were saying
- Using incorrect or vague words

Over time, the person may begin to avoid conversations.

This is often due to frustration or embarrassment.

Personality and Mood Changes

Sometimes, the earliest sign is not memory loss, but a change in personality.

A person may become:

- Irritable or easily upset
- Suspicious or fearful
- Withdrawn from social interactions
- Less interested in activities they once enjoyed

Families often say, "This is not how they used to be."

That observation is important.

Early Warning Signs of Dementia

❶ Memory Loss

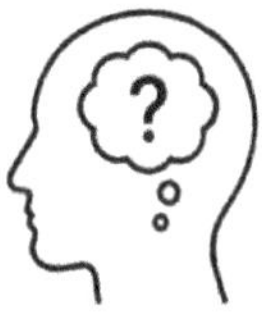

- Forgets recent events
- Repeats questions

❷ Difficulty Planning

- Trouble organizing tasks
- Struggles with decisions

❸ Getting Lost

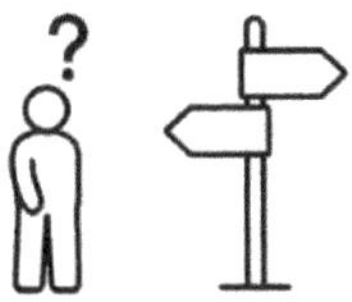

- Confused in familiar places
- Loses direction

❹ Language Problems

- Difficulty finding words
- Pauses while speaking

❺ Behavior Changes

- Irritability
- Withdrawal

❻ Daily Tasks Become Difficult

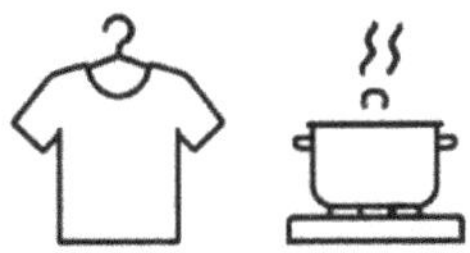

- Trouble with routine work
- Needs reminders

Early changes affect daily life and should not be ignored

Difficulty Performing Familiar Tasks

Routine activities may slowly become challenging.

You may notice:

- Trouble cooking familiar meals
- Difficulty managing medications
- Problems handling money
- Neglect of personal care

These changes usually develop gradually, but they become more noticeable over time.

Loss of Initiative and Interest

A person may lose motivation.

They may:

- Sit quietly for long periods
- Avoid social interaction
- Show less interest in daily life

This is not laziness.

It is part of the disease process affecting the brain.

A Real-Life Reflection

A 71-year-old woman who had always been active began avoiding social gatherings.

Her family noticed she was repeating stories and occasionally forgetting recent conversations.

Later, she became confused while driving to a familiar place.

At first, the family thought this was normal aging.

But the pattern became clear over time.

She was evaluated and diagnosed with early dementia.

Because the signs were recognized, her family was able to plan early and provide better support.

Doctor's Pearl

Early warning signs are often subtle but consistent. When changes begin to affect daily life, they should not be ignored.

Myth vs Fact

Myth: If a person can speak normally, their memory is fine.

Fact: Early dementia can be present even when speech appears normal. Subtle changes in memory and judgment may already exist.

Common Mistakes to Avoid

- Ignoring repeated symptoms
- Assuming changes are due to aging
- Delaying medical evaluation
- Arguing with the patient instead of observing patterns

Red Flag Warnings

- Frequent repetition of questions
- Getting lost in familiar surroundings
- Unsafe decisions, especially financial or driving-related
- Noticeable personality changes

Chapter Summary

Early warning signs of dementia are gradual and subtle.
Memory loss is only one part of the condition.
Changes in thinking, behavior, and daily function are equally important.
Recognizing patterns early allows timely evaluation and better planning.

Action Plan

- Observe and document repeated changes
- Discuss concerns openly within the family
- Seek medical evaluation if symptoms persist
- Pay attention to safety-related issues
- Trust your instincts when something feels different

Transition to Next Chapter

Now that we have clearly identified the early warning signs, the next step is to understand Mild Cognitive Impairment, a stage where changes are present but independence is still largely maintained, and where early action can make a meaningful difference.

CHAPTER 4: Mild Cognitive Impairment – The Critical Window We Should Not Miss

The Stage That Lies Between Normal Aging and Dementia

In many patients, dementia does not begin suddenly.

There is often a phase in between. A stage where something is not quite right, but life is still largely manageable.

This stage is called **Mild Cognitive Impairment**, or MCI.

It is one of the most important stages in the entire journey of dementia.

Because this is the stage where we still have time.

Time to understand what is happening.
Time to act.
Time to influence what comes next.

What Exactly Is Mild Cognitive Impairment

Mild Cognitive Impairment is a condition where there is a noticeable decline in memory or thinking ability, but daily functioning is mostly preserved.

A person with MCI may:

- Forget recent conversations
- Misplace things more often
- Take longer to complete familiar tasks
- Need reminders more frequently

But importantly, they can still:

- Live independently
- Manage basic daily activities
- Handle most routine responsibilities

This is the key difference.

In dementia, independence begins to decline.
In MCI, independence is largely maintained.

Why This Stage Is So Important

Many families either miss this stage or do not take it seriously.

They may say, "It is not severe yet."

But this is exactly the stage where attention matters the most.

At this point:

- The patient is often aware of changes
- Decisions can still be made clearly
- Lifestyle changes can be implemented
- Medical evaluation can identify reversible causes

If we act here, we can often slow progression or stabilize the condition.

If we ignore it, we lose that opportunity.

Different Types of Mild Cognitive Impairment

Not all MCI is the same.

There are two main patterns:

Amnestic MCI

- Memory is the main problem
- Higher risk of progressing to Alzheimer-type dementia

Non-amnestic MCI

- Problems with attention, language, or thinking
- May progress to other types of dementia

Recognizing the pattern helps guide follow-up and planning.

Will It Progress to Dementia

This is one of the most common questions.

The answer is not the same for everyone.

Some people with MCI:

- Remain stable for years
- Improve when underlying causes are treated
- Gradually progress to dementia

There is no fixed rule.

However, MCI does increase the risk of future dementia.

That is why monitoring is essential.

Reversible and Contributing Factors That Must Be Checked

One of the most important parts of evaluation is identifying conditions that can worsen memory.

These include:

- Medication side effects
- Depression and anxiety
- Sleep disorders such as sleep apnea
- Vitamin B12 deficiency
- Thyroid problems
- Alcohol use

- Hearing and vision impairment

Addressing these can lead to improvement or stabilization.

This step should never be skipped.

Doctor's Pearl

Before labeling someone with progressive cognitive decline, always look for reversible causes. This can make a meaningful difference.

Monitoring and Follow-Up

MCI is not a one-time diagnosis.

It requires ongoing observation.

Patients should be followed regularly for:

- Changes in memory or thinking
- Ability to perform daily tasks
- New behavioral or functional changes

This helps detect progression early and adjust care.

The Emotional Impact at This Stage

This stage can be emotionally difficult.

The patient is often aware of the changes.

They may feel:

- Worried about the future
- Frustrated with themselves
- Anxious about losing independence

Families may feel uncertain.

Is this serious? Will it progress?

Open communication and reassurance are very important at this stage.

A Real-Life Reflection

A 66-year-old man noticed that he was taking longer to complete routine tasks.

He also began forgetting recent discussions.

He was evaluated and diagnosed with Mild Cognitive Impairment.

Further evaluation revealed untreated sleep apnea and mild depression.

With treatment, improved sleep, and lifestyle changes, his symptoms stabilized.

Several years later, he remained independent.

This is the value of early recognition.

Myth vs Fact

Myth: Mild Cognitive Impairment always leads to dementia.
Fact: Many individuals with MCI remain stable or improve, especially when contributing factors are addressed.

Common Mistakes to Avoid

- Ignoring early symptoms
- Assuming MCI is harmless
- Not evaluating reversible causes
- Skipping regular follow-up

Red Flag Warnings

- Rapid worsening of symptoms
- Loss of independence in daily activities
- New personality or behavioral changes
- Safety concerns such as getting lost

Chapter Summary

Mild Cognitive Impairment is a stage between normal aging and dementia.
Memory or thinking problems are present, but independence is largely preserved.
Not all cases progress to dementia.
Reversible causes must always be evaluated.
Early recognition allows better planning and management.

Action Plan

- Seek evaluation for persistent cognitive changes
- Review medications and medical conditions
- Address sleep, mood, and nutritional factors
- Stay physically, mentally, and socially active
- Schedule regular follow-up

Transition to Next Chapter

Now that we understand this important middle stage, the next step is to explore the different causes and types of dementia, so that we can better understand how and why these changes develop in the brain.

CHAPTER 5: The Major Types of Dementia – Understanding the Differences That Matter

One Word, Many Diseases

When families hear the word "dementia," they often think it is one single illness.

In reality, dementia is a broad term. It describes a pattern of symptoms, not one disease.

Under this umbrella are several conditions. Each has its own cause, its own pattern, and its own course over time.

Why does this matter?

Because understanding the type helps you:

- Know what to expect
- Recognize symptoms early
- Avoid unnecessary confusion
- Make better decisions about care

Clarity at this stage makes the journey ahead more manageable.

Alzheimer’s disease: The Most Common Form

This is the most common cause of dementia.

It usually begins slowly.

Early symptoms often include:

- Difficulty remembering recent events
- Repeating questions
- Misplacing items

As the condition progresses, it affects:

- Language
- Judgment
- Daily functioning

The decline is generally gradual and continuous.

Families often describe it as a slow fading of memory and independence.

Vascular Dementia – When Blood Flow Is Affected

Vascular dementia occurs when blood supply to the brain is reduced.

This may happen due to:

- Stroke
- Small vessel disease
- Long-standing high blood pressure
- Diabetes or high cholesterol

Unlike Alzheimer-type dementia, the decline may not be smooth.

It may appear:

- Suddenly after a stroke
- In a stepwise pattern, with periods of stability followed by decline

Common features include:

- Slowed thinking
- Difficulty planning and organizing
- Problems with attention

Controlling vascular risk factors is very important in this type.

Lewy Body Dementia – A Distinct Pattern

Lewy body dementia has some unique features.

Patients may experience:

- Visual hallucinations, often early
- Fluctuating alertness

- Parkinson-like symptoms such as stiffness or slow movement

Memory loss may not be the first symptom.

One important point is sensitivity to certain medications, especially some antipsychotic drugs.

Recognizing this type early can help prevent complications.

Frontotemporal Dementia – When Behavior Changes First

This type often affects younger individuals compared to other dementias.

The early signs are usually not memory-related.

Families may notice:

- Personality changes
- Loss of social judgment
- Impulsive or inappropriate behavior
- Reduced empathy

In some cases, language problems are more prominent.

Because memory may be relatively preserved early, diagnosis is often delayed.

Parkinson's Disease Dementia

In patients with Parkinson's disease, cognitive decline may develop over time.

Features may include:

- Slowed thinking
- Difficulty with attention
- Visual hallucinations

This typically occurs after years of movement-related symptoms.

Understanding the connection helps guide treatment decisions.

Mixed Dementia – More Than One Cause

In many older adults, more than one type of brain change occurs.

The most common combination includes:

- Alzheimer-type changes
- Vascular changes

This is called mixed dementia.

It is very common in real-world practice.

Symptoms may overlap, making diagnosis less straightforward.

Why Identifying the Type Matters

Some families ask, “Does it really matter which type it is?”

The answer is yes.

Knowing the type helps:

- Guide treatment decisions
- Anticipate symptoms
- Avoid certain medications
- Plan care more effectively

Even though there is overlap, understanding the likely cause brings clarity.

A Real-Life Reflection

A 72-year-old man began experiencing vivid visual hallucinations.

He described seeing people in the room who were not there.

At the same time, his alertness varied from day to day.

Initially, this was thought to be a psychiatric issue.

Further evaluation revealed Lewy body dementia.

Once the correct diagnosis was made, unnecessary medications were avoided, and his care improved.

This highlights the importance of accurate diagnosis.

Doctor's Pearl

Different types of dementia may look similar at first, but their patterns and management can be very different. A careful diagnosis always helps.

Myth vs Fact

Myth: All dementia is Alzheimer's disease.
Fact: Alzheimer's is the most common cause, but several other diseases can lead to dementia.

Common Mistakes to Avoid

- Assuming all dementia behaves the same way
- Ignoring unusual symptoms such as hallucinations
- Delaying specialist evaluation when needed
- Using medications without a clear diagnosis

Red Flag Warnings

- Early hallucinations
- Sudden or stepwise decline
- Marked personality change
- Movement problems along with cognitive decline

Chapter Summary

Dementia can be caused by several different diseases. Alzheimer's disease is the most common, but not the only cause.
Each type has distinct features and progression patterns. Understanding the type helps guide treatment and planning.

Action Plan

- Seek proper evaluation to identify the likely type
- Observe and report specific symptoms clearly
- Control blood pressure, diabetes, and cholesterol
- Ask questions to understand the diagnosis
- Do not assume all dementia is the same

Transition to Next Chapter

Now that we understand the major types of dementia, the next step is to explore conditions that can mimic dementia and may be reversible, so that treatable causes are not missed.

CHAPTER 6: Memory Loss That May Be Reversible – Do Not Miss These Treatable Causes

Before We Call It Dementia, We Must Be Careful

When a patient comes with memory problems, one of the most important responsibilities as a physician is this:

Do not rush to label it as dementia.

Because not all memory loss is permanent.

Not all confusion means progressive brain disease.

In fact, many conditions can **mimic dementia**, and some of them are **treatable and reversible**.

Missing these conditions can lead to unnecessary fear and missed opportunities for recovery.

Recognizing them early can completely change the outcome.

Why This Step Matters So Much

If a reversible cause is overlooked:

- The patient may be wrongly labeled
- The family may lose hope unnecessarily
- Treatment may be delayed
- The condition may worsen unnecessarily

On the other hand, identifying a reversible cause can:

- Improve memory and thinking
- Restore function
- Reduce anxiety for both patient and family

This is why a careful evaluation is essential in every case.

Medications – A Common and Often Missed Cause

One of the most frequent causes of memory problems is medication.

Many commonly used drugs can affect brain function, especially in older adults.

These include:

- Sleeping pills
- Anti-anxiety medications
- Certain pain medications
- Antihistamines
- Some bladder medications
- Older antidepressants

As the brain ages, it becomes more sensitive to these effects.

Sometimes, simply adjusting or stopping a medication leads to noticeable improvement.

Doctor's Pearl

Always review medications in any patient with memory concerns. This is one of the most correctable causes of cognitive problems.

Depression – When Mood Affects Memory

Depression can closely resemble dementia.

Patients may:

- Complain of poor memory
- Have difficulty concentrating
- Appear withdrawn
- Show lack of interest

This is sometimes called "pseudodementia."

The important difference is that cognitive function often improves when depression is treated.

This highlights how closely emotional health and brain function are connected.

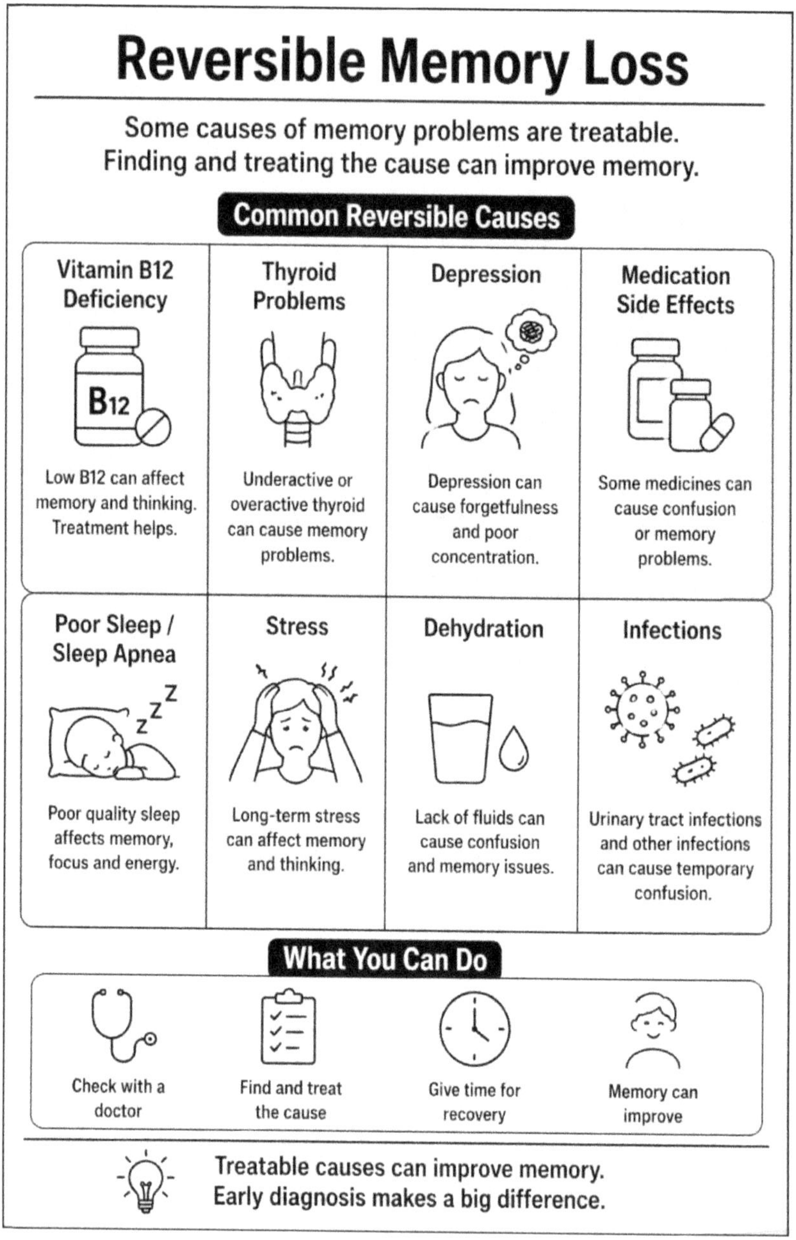
Reversible Memory Loss
Some causes of memory problems are treatable.
Finding and treating the cause can improve memory.
Common Reversible Causes
Vitamin B12 Deficiency
B12
Low B12 can affect memory and thinking. Treatment helps.
Thyroid Problems
Underactive or overactive thyroid can cause memory problems.
Depression
Depression can cause forgetfulness and poor concentration.
Medication Side Effects
Some medicines can cause confusion or memory problems.
Poor Sleep / Sleep Apnea
Z Z Z
Poor quality sleep affects memory, focus and energy.
Stress
Long-term stress can affect memory and thinking.
Dehydration
Lack of fluids can cause confusion and memory issues.
Infections
Urinary tract infections and other infections can cause temporary confusion.
What You Can Do
Check with a doctor
Find and treat the cause
Give time for recovery
Memory can improve
Treatable causes can improve memory.
Early diagnosis makes a big difference.

Sleep Disorders – The Hidden Contributor

Sleep is essential for brain function.

Conditions such as sleep apnea are very common and often undiagnosed.

They can lead to:

- Daytime fatigue
- Poor concentration
- Memory problems
- Irritability

Treating sleep disorders can lead to significant improvement.

Good sleep is not optional. It is essential for brain health.

Vitamin Deficiencies and Hormonal Problems

Certain medical conditions can directly affect cognition.

Important ones include:

- Vitamin B12 deficiency
- Thyroid disorders
- Electrolyte imbalances

These are often detected through simple blood tests.

When corrected, memory and thinking may improve.

Delirium – A Medical Emergency

In older adults, sudden confusion should always be taken seriously.

This condition is called **delirium**.

It often develops quickly and may fluctuate.

Common causes include:

- Infections such as urinary tract infections or pneumonia
- Medication changes
- Dehydration
- Acute illness

Unlike dementia, delirium is often reversible if treated promptly.

This is why sudden confusion is a medical emergency.

Alcohol and Substance Use

Excessive alcohol use can impair memory and thinking.

Over time, it may lead to long-term brain damage.

Even moderate alcohol use, especially when combined with medications, can worsen cognitive function.

Reducing or stopping alcohol may improve symptoms in some cases.

Hearing and Vision Problems

This is often overlooked.

When a person cannot hear or see well:

- Conversations become difficult
- Social interaction decreases
- Confusion increases

The brain has to work harder to compensate.

Correcting hearing and vision problems can significantly improve daily functioning.

Dehydration and General Health

Something as simple as dehydration can affect mental clarity, especially in older adults.

Other factors such as poor nutrition, chronic illness, and fatigue can also contribute.

Improving overall health often leads to better cognitive function.

A Real-Life Reflection

A 69-year-old woman was brought in with memory loss and confusion.

Her family feared dementia.

On evaluation, she was found to have:

- Severe vitamin B12 deficiency
- Poor sleep due to untreated sleep apnea
- Medications affecting cognition

With treatment and adjustment, her memory improved significantly over a few months.

This case highlights an important lesson.

Not all memory loss is permanent.

Myth vs Fact

Myth: Memory loss in older age always means dementia.
Fact: Many medical and psychological conditions can cause memory problems, and some are reversible.

Common Mistakes to Avoid

- Jumping to a diagnosis without proper evaluation
- Ignoring medication effects
- Overlooking depression or sleep disorders
- Delaying medical attention for sudden confusion

Red Flag Warnings

- Sudden onset of confusion
- Rapid fluctuation in alertness
- New symptoms after starting a medication
- Significant decline during illness

Chapter Summary

Not all memory problems are due to dementia.
Several conditions can mimic or worsen cognitive decline.
Many of these causes are treatable or reversible.
A thorough evaluation is essential before making a diagnosis.

Action Plan

- Review all medications with your doctor
- Get basic blood tests including B12 and thyroid function
- Address sleep problems and emotional health

- Seek urgent care for sudden confusion
- Do not assume the worst without proper evaluation

Transition to Next Chapter

Now that we understand that some causes of memory loss may be reversible, the next step is to explore risk factors for dementia and what we can do to protect brain health over time.

CHAPTER 7: Risk Factors and Brain Protection – What You Can Still Control

A Question Almost Everyone Asks

Sooner or later, this question comes.

“Doctor, can this be prevented?”

It is a simple question, but the answer requires a balanced and honest response.

We cannot prevent all cases of dementia. Age and genetics do play a role.

But we are not helpless.

A significant part of the risk is influenced by factors we can understand and manage.

This chapter is not about fear.

It is about control, awareness, and long-term protection.

Two Types of Risk – What We Can and Cannot Change

To understand prevention, we must first understand risk.

There are two broad categories.

Non-modifiable risk factors

- Increasing age
- Family history
- Genetic factors

These cannot be changed.

Modifiable risk factors

- High blood pressure
- Diabetes
- High cholesterol
- Obesity
- Smoking
- Physical inactivity
- Poor diet
- Sleep disorders
- Depression
- Social isolation
- Hearing loss

This is where we can make a meaningful difference.

Doctor's Pearl

Dementia prevention is not about one dramatic change. It is about steady, consistent habits over time.

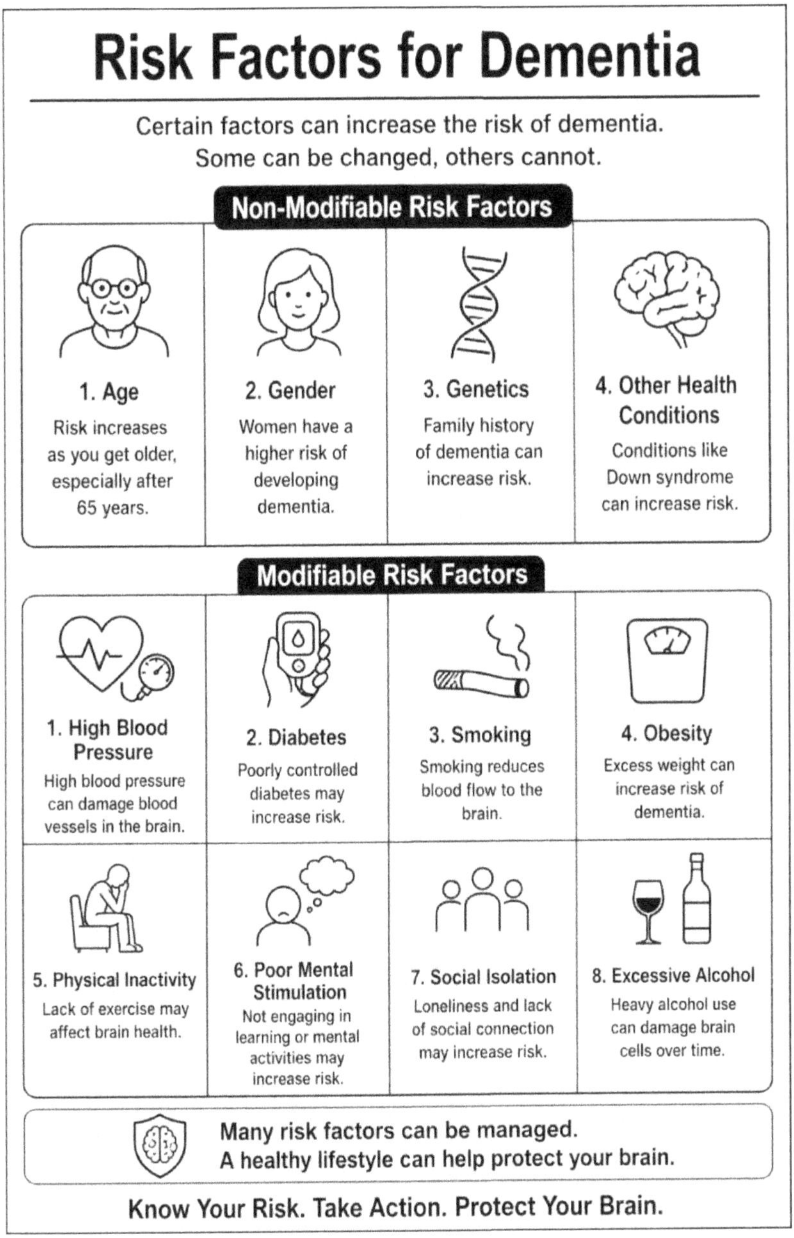
Risk Factors for Dementia
Certain factors can increase the risk of dementia.
Some can be changed, others cannot.
Non-Modifiable Risk Factors
1. Age
Risk increases as you get older, especially after 65 years.
2. Gender
Women have a higher risk of developing dementia.
3. Genetics
Family history of dementia can increase risk.
4. Other Health Conditions
Conditions like Down syndrome can increase risk.
Modifiable Risk Factors
1. High Blood Pressure
High blood pressure can damage blood vessels in the brain.
2. Diabetes
Poorly controlled diabetes may increase risk.
3. Smoking
Smoking reduces blood flow to the brain.
4. Obesity
Excess weight can increase risk of dementia.
5. Physical Inactivity
Lack of exercise may affect brain health.
6. Poor Mental Stimulation
Not engaging in learning or mental activities may increase risk.
7. Social Isolation
Loneliness and lack of social connection may increase risk.
8. Excessive Alcohol
Heavy alcohol use can damage brain cells over time.
Many risk factors can be managed.
A healthy lifestyle can help protect your brain.
Know Your Risk. Take Action. Protect Your Brain.

The Brain and Blood Flow – A Critical Link

The brain depends on a steady, healthy blood supply.

Conditions such as:

- High blood pressure
- Diabetes
- High cholesterol

damage blood vessels over time.

This reduces blood flow to the brain and increases the risk of cognitive decline.

Managing these conditions is one of the most effective ways to protect brain health.

Regular follow-up and proper treatment are essential.

Physical Activity – A Powerful Tool

Regular movement supports brain health in several ways.

It helps:

- Improve blood circulation

- Maintain overall health
- Enhance mood
- Support better sleep

You do not need intense exercise.

Simple activities such as:

- Brisk walking
- Light exercises
- Daily movement

can make a meaningful difference.

Consistency is more important than intensity.

Nutrition – Feeding the Brain Properly

What we eat influences how our brain functions.

A balanced diet should include:

- Fruits and vegetables
- Whole grains
- Nuts and seeds
- Fish and healthy fats

At the same time, it is important to reduce:

- Processed foods
- Excess sugar

- Unhealthy fats

Healthy eating supports both brain and overall health.

Sleep – The Brain's Maintenance System

Sleep is essential for memory and brain function.

During sleep:

- The brain processes information
- Waste products are cleared

Poor sleep can lead to:

- Reduced concentration
- Memory problems
- Increased long-term risk

Conditions such as sleep apnea should be identified and treated.

Mental Activity – Keep the Brain Engaged

The brain benefits from regular use.

Helpful activities include:

- Reading
- Learning new skills
- Playing games
- Solving puzzles

It is not about complexity.

It is about staying engaged regularly.

Social Connection – More Important Than We Think

Human connection plays a significant role in brain health.

Isolation can worsen both mood and cognition.

Regular interaction with:

- Family
- Friends
- Community

helps maintain emotional and mental well-being.

Even simple conversations matter.

Hearing and Vision – Often Overlooked

Hearing loss is strongly associated with cognitive decline.

When hearing is impaired:

- Communication becomes difficult
- Social interaction decreases
- The brain works harder to process sound

Using hearing aids when needed can help reduce this strain.

Similarly, correcting vision problems improves overall functioning.

Avoiding Harmful Habits

Certain habits increase risk.

These include:

- Smoking
- Excess alcohol use
- Sedentary lifestyle

Reducing or eliminating these habits improves overall health and brain function.

A Real-Life Reflection

A 62-year-old man with high blood pressure and diabetes became concerned about his memory.

He made gradual changes:

- Improved diet
- Regular walking
- Better sleep
- Strict control of his medical conditions

Over time, his overall health improved, and his cognitive concerns stabilized.

This is not uncommon.

Small, consistent steps can make a meaningful difference.

Myth vs Fact

Myth: Nothing can be done to prevent dementia.
Fact: Many risk factors can be modified, and addressing them can reduce or delay the risk.

Common Mistakes to Avoid

- Waiting until symptoms appear before taking action
- Ignoring chronic medical conditions
- Underestimating the importance of sleep
- Neglecting social engagement

Red Flag Warnings

- Uncontrolled blood pressure or diabetes
- Severe sleep problems
- Increasing social withdrawal
- Untreated hearing loss

Chapter Summary

Dementia risk is influenced by both modifiable and non-modifiable factors.
Many risks can be reduced through lifestyle and medical management.
Exercise, diet, sleep, and social engagement are essential.
Long-term consistency is the key to brain protection.

Action Plan

- Keep blood pressure, diabetes, and cholesterol under control
- Engage in regular physical activity
- Follow a balanced, healthy diet
- Maintain good sleep habits
- Stay mentally and socially active
- Address hearing and vision problems
- Avoid smoking and limit alcohol

Transition to Next Chapter

Now that we understand how to protect brain health and reduce risk, the next step is to understand how dementia is diagnosed, so that concerns can be evaluated clearly and accurately.

CHAPTER 8: How Dementia Is Diagnosed – From Doubt to Clarity

When It Is Time to Seek Answers

By the time families reach this stage, something has already changed.

What began as a few small doubts has become a clear concern.

Something feels different. The pattern is no longer occasional. It is becoming consistent.

This is the point where many families decide to seek medical advice.

And this step, though sometimes delayed, is one of the most important in the entire journey.

Diagnosis is not about labeling a person.

It is about understanding what is happening, why it is happening, and what should be done next.

Clarity at this stage reduces confusion, fear, and unnecessary delay.

The Most Important Tool – A Careful History

In dementia evaluation, the most valuable information often comes from listening.

Doctors will carefully ask:

- When did the symptoms begin
- How have they changed over time
- What specific problems have been noticed
- How daily life has been affected

Family members play a critical role.

In many cases, the patient may not recognize or remember the changes.

This is why input from a spouse or close relative is essential.

Doctor's Pearl

In dementia diagnosis, the patient's story and the family's observations are often more important than any single test.

Cognitive Testing – Understanding Brain Function

Doctors use structured tests to evaluate different areas of thinking.

These include:

- Memory
- Attention
- Language
- Problem-solving
- Orientation

Some tests are brief and used for screening.

Others are more detailed and provide deeper assessment.

These tests help:

- Detect cognitive impairment
- Understand the pattern of deficits
- Estimate the severity

They are an important part of evaluation, but they do not stand alone.

Physical and Neurological Examination

A careful examination helps identify other possible causes.

Doctors look for:

- Signs of stroke
- Movement problems
- Balance issues
- Sensory changes

This helps differentiate between types of dementia and other neurological conditions.

Laboratory Tests – Looking for Treatable Causes

Blood tests are essential.

They help detect:

- Vitamin B12 deficiency
- Thyroid disorders
- Electrolyte imbalances
- Infections

These conditions can mimic or worsen cognitive problems.

Identifying them early can lead to improvement.

Medication Review – A Critical Step

Many patients take multiple medications.

Some of these can affect memory and thinking.

Doctors will review:

- Prescription medications
- Over-the-counter drugs
- Supplements

Adjusting medications can sometimes improve symptoms significantly.

Brain Imaging – Looking Inside the Brain

Imaging studies such as CT scan or MRI are commonly used.

They help identify:

- Stroke or vascular changes
- Brain atrophy
- Tumors or structural abnormalities

MRI provides more detailed information when needed.

Imaging does not always give a complete diagnosis, but it provides important clues.

How is Dementia Diagnosed?

Dementia is diagnosed through a careful evaluation of symptoms, tests and medical history.

1 Medical History and Interview

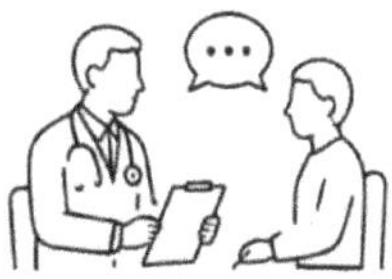

The doctor asks about memory problems, other symptoms, medical history, medications and changes in daily life.

2 Cognitive and Memory Tests

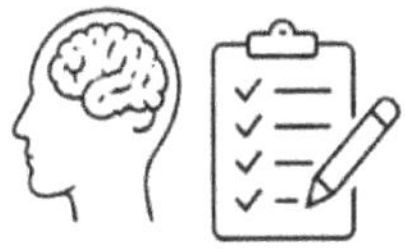

Simple tests check memory, attention, language, problem solving and other thinking skills.

3 Physical and Neurological Exam

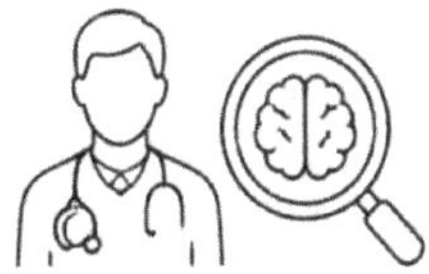

The doctor examines general health, nerves, reflexes, movement, balance and other functions.

4 Laboratory Tests

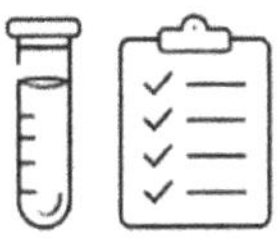

Blood and urine tests find problems like vitamin deficiency, thyroid issues, infections or other conditions that can affect memory.

5 Brain Imaging

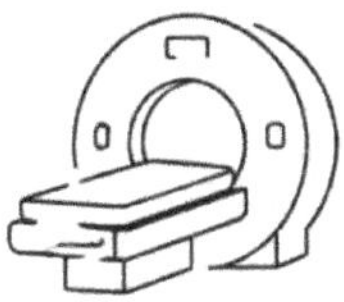

MRI or CT scan shows changes in the brain and helps rule out other causes of memory problems.

6 Other Tests (If Needed)

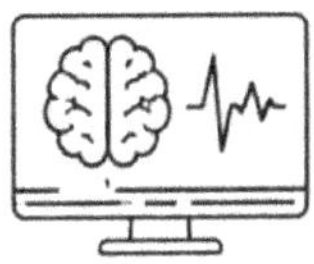

Tests like EEG or PET scan may be used in certain cases to get more information.

7 Review and Diagnosis

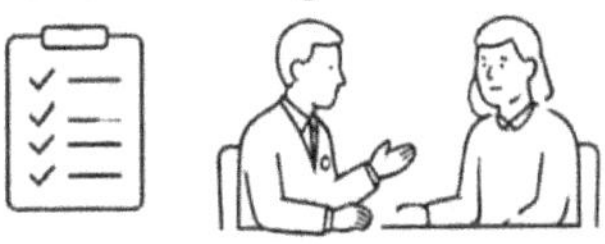

The doctor reviews all findings and decides if symptoms are due to dementia or another treatable condition.

Early and accurate diagnosis helps in better treatment, planning and support for a better quality of life.

When Specialist Evaluation Is Needed

In some cases, referral to a specialist is helpful.

This may include:

- Neurologists
- Geriatricians
- Memory clinics

Specialists may perform advanced testing or provide more detailed assessment.

This is especially useful when:

- The diagnosis is unclear
- Symptoms are unusual
- The patient is relatively young

Why Diagnosis Is Not Always Immediate

Families often expect a clear answer after one visit.

In reality, diagnosis may take time.

Reasons include:

- Overlapping symptoms between conditions
- Presence of multiple contributing factors

- Early-stage subtle changes
- Coexisting depression or delirium

Follow-up and reassessment are often necessary.

Diagnosis is a process, not a single event.

A Real-Life Reflection

A 70-year-old man presented with memory concerns.

Initial evaluation suggested mild cognitive impairment.

Blood tests revealed vitamin B12 deficiency. Imaging showed small vessel changes.

With treatment and better control of his medical conditions, his symptoms stabilized.

This case illustrates an important point.

Diagnosis is often a combination of factors, not a single finding.

Myth vs Fact

Myth: A single test can diagnose dementia.
Fact: Diagnosis requires a combination of history, examination, tests, and follow-up.

Common Mistakes to Avoid

- Delaying evaluation
- Providing incomplete history
- Ignoring medication effects
- Expecting immediate answers

Red Flag Warnings

- Rapid decline over weeks or months
- Sudden confusion
- New neurological symptoms
- Significant change after starting a medication

Chapter Summary

Diagnosis of dementia is a structured and careful process.
History from patient and family is essential.
Cognitive testing, examination, lab tests, and imaging all play a role.
Reversible causes must always be evaluated.
Diagnosis often requires time and follow-up.

Action Plan

- Seek medical evaluation if concerns persist
- Prepare a clear history before the visit
- Bring a family member for additional input
- Review medications carefully
- Follow up regularly

Transition to Next Chapter

Now that we understand how dementia is diagnosed, the next step is to explore newer tests and biomarkers that are changing how we detect and understand dementia in modern medicine.

CHAPTER 9: New Tests, Biomarkers, and the Future of Diagnosis

A New Era in Understanding Dementia

For many years, diagnosing dementia depended mainly on clinical judgment.

Doctors relied on history, examination, and basic tests. That approach is still the foundation of good care.

But medicine is evolving.

Today, we are beginning to look deeper into the brain. Not just at its structure, but at the disease process itself.

This has led to the development of **biomarkers**, tools that can detect early changes in the brain long before symptoms become obvious.

This progress is exciting.

It offers the possibility of earlier diagnosis, better understanding, and more targeted treatment.

At the same time, it requires careful interpretation.

What Are Biomarkers and Why Do They Matter

A biomarker is a measurable sign of disease.

In dementia, especially Alzheimer-type conditions, biomarkers help detect:

- Abnormal protein accumulation
- Early disease activity
- Changes in brain function

These changes may begin years before symptoms appear.

This has two important implications:

- Earlier identification of disease
- Better selection of patients for newer treatments

However, biomarkers are supportive tools.

They do not replace careful clinical evaluation.

Amyloid and Tau – The Key Proteins

In Alzheimer-type dementia, two proteins play a central role:

- Amyloid
- Tau

These proteins accumulate abnormally in the brain.

Over time, they interfere with normal brain function and lead to damage of brain cells.

Detecting these proteins can support the diagnosis.

However, it is important to understand:

The presence of these proteins does not always mean that a person will develop symptoms.

This is why interpretation must always be done in clinical context.

PET Scans – Looking Beyond Structure

Positron Emission Tomography, or PET scan, is an advanced imaging technique.

It can:

- Detect amyloid deposits
- Assess brain metabolism
- Help differentiate types of dementia

PET scans can provide valuable information in selected cases.

However:

- They are expensive
- Not widely available everywhere
- Not required for routine diagnosis

They are best used when the diagnosis is uncertain or when advanced treatment decisions are being considered.

Cerebrospinal Fluid Testing

Another method involves analyzing cerebrospinal fluid through a lumbar puncture.

This test measures:

- Amyloid levels
- Tau protein levels

Changes in these markers can support the diagnosis of Alzheimer-type dementia.

While useful, this test is invasive and is not required in all patients.

Blood Tests – A Promising Development

One of the most exciting recent developments is the emergence of blood-based tests.

These tests aim to detect biomarkers such as amyloid and tau in the blood.

Potential advantages include:

- Less invasive
- Easier to perform
- More accessible

However, these tests are still evolving.

They are not yet a simple yes-or-no answer for dementia.

They must be interpreted carefully along with clinical findings.

Doctor's Pearl

Advanced tests can support diagnosis, but they never replace careful clinical judgment. The patient's history remains the foundation.

Who Should Consider Advanced Testing

Not every patient needs these tests.

They may be useful when:

- The diagnosis is unclear

- Symptoms are unusual
- Early-stage disease needs confirmation
- New treatments are being considered

In many routine cases, standard evaluation is sufficient.

Limitations and Cautions

While these tests are promising, they have limitations.

- They are not perfect
- Abnormal results may be seen in people without symptoms
- They can create anxiety if misunderstood
- Cost and availability may be barriers

Over-reliance on tests without clinical context can lead to confusion.

A Real-Life Reflection

A 64-year-old patient presented with mild memory concerns.

Initial evaluation suggested early Alzheimer-type changes, but there was uncertainty.

Advanced imaging confirmed amyloid deposition.

This helped guide further management and allowed consideration of newer therapies.

However, the final diagnosis still depended on the overall clinical picture.

Myth vs Fact

Myth: A blood test can definitively diagnose dementia.
Fact: Blood tests can support diagnosis, but they are not standalone tools.

Common Mistakes to Avoid

- Assuming advanced tests are always necessary
- Relying only on test results
- Misinterpreting results without medical guidance
- Seeking tests without a clear purpose

Red Flag Warnings

- Unusual or rapidly progressing symptoms
- Early onset of cognitive decline
- Conflicting findings from standard evaluation
- Strong family history with unclear diagnosis

New and Future Tests for Dementia

Research is improving how we detect dementia earlier and more accurately. These tests are new or under development.

NEW TESTS (Available or in Some Centers)

1. Biomarker Blood Tests

- Detect proteins linked to Alzheimer's (e.g., amyloid, tau).
- Simple blood test in the future.
- Helps in early diagnosis.

2. Amyloid PET Scan

- Detects amyloid plaques in the brain.
- Useful for early Alzheimer's detection.
- More accurate diagnosis.

3. Tau PET Scan

- Detects tau tangles in the brain.
- Shows how much damage has occurred.
- Helps in disease progression.

4. Advanced MRI

- High-resolution MRI shows changes in brain structure.
- Detects shrinkage in specific areas early.
- Tracks progression.

FUTURE TESTS (Under Research)

5. Genetic Testing

- Identifies genes that may increase risk.
- Helps in personalized risk assessment and prevention.
- Useful for family planning.

6. Digital Biomarkers

- Uses data from memory games, voice, typing, sleep and activity.
- Detects subtle changes over time.
- Can alert early before symptoms.

7. Eye Scan (Retinal Imaging)

- Examines tiny blood vessels in the retina.
- May show early signs of brain changes.
- Fast, non-invasive and painless.

8. Advanced AI-Based Tests

- Artificial intelligence analyzes multiple tests and data.
- Improves accuracy in early detection and prediction.
- Supports better decisions.

These new and future tests aim for earlier detection, more accurate diagnosis and better care for patients.

Research today, better brain health tomorrow.

Chapter Summary

Biomarkers are changing how dementia is diagnosed.
Amyloid and tau proteins are central in Alzheimer-type disease.
Advanced tests include PET scans, cerebrospinal fluid analysis, and emerging blood tests.
These tests are useful in selected cases but do not replace clinical evaluation.
Careful interpretation is essential.

Action Plan

- Discuss with your doctor whether advanced testing is needed
- Understand the purpose and limitations of each test
- Avoid relying on tests alone
- Use results as part of a broader clinical picture
- Stay informed about ongoing developments

Transition to Next Chapter

Now that we understand how modern testing is shaping diagnosis, the next step is to understand how dementia progresses over time, so families can prepare for each stage with clarity and confidence.

CHAPTER 10: Understanding the Stages of Dementia – What to Expect, What to Do

A Journey That Unfolds Gradually

One of the most difficult parts of dementia is uncertainty.

Families often ask, "What will happen next?"

There is no single timeline that applies to everyone. Each person's journey is different.

But in most cases, dementia follows a general pattern. It progresses slowly, over time, in stages.

Understanding these stages does not remove the difficulty.

But it does something very important.

It replaces uncertainty with clarity.

And when families know what to expect, they are better prepared to respond with patience, planning, and confidence.

Why Understanding Stages Matters

Knowing the stages helps in practical ways.

It allows families to:

- Plan ahead
- Recognize changes early
- Adjust care appropriately
- Set realistic expectations

It also reduces frustration.

When you understand that a behavior is part of the stage, you are less likely to take it personally.

The Early Stage – Subtle but Important

This is where the journey usually begins.

Symptoms may be mild and easy to overlook.

Common features include:

- Forgetting recent conversations
- Repeating questions
- Difficulty finding words
- Losing track of time
- Mild problems with planning

At this stage, most patients remain independent.

They can:

- Live on their own
- Drive
- Manage finances

However, tasks may take more effort.

Emotionally, this stage can be difficult.

Patients may feel:

- Frustrated
- Anxious
- Embarrassed

They are often aware of their difficulties.

Doctor's Pearl

The early stage is the best time to plan ahead. Decisions made now can prevent stress later.

The Middle Stage – Increasing Dependence

As the disease progresses, changes become more noticeable.

Memory problems worsen.

New symptoms may include:

- Confusion about time and place
- Difficulty recognizing familiar people
- Problems with language
- Behavioral changes such as agitation or suspicion

Daily activities become more challenging.

Patients may need help with:

- Cooking
- Managing medications
- Dressing
- Personal care

Safety becomes a major concern.

Families may notice:

- Wandering
- Sleep disturbances
- Repetitive behaviors

This stage often lasts the longest and requires increasing caregiver involvement.

The Late Stage – Complete Dependence

In the advanced stage, the impact is significant.

Patients may:

- Lose the ability to communicate clearly
- Become unable to recognize loved ones
- Have difficulty swallowing
- Lose mobility

They become fully dependent on others.

Other concerns may include:

- Weight loss
- Infections
- Incontinence

At this stage, care focuses on comfort, dignity, and quality of life.

Functional Decline – Beyond Memory

Dementia affects more than memory.

Over time, it impacts:

- Physical strength
- Balance
- Coordination
- Ability to perform basic tasks

This leads to increasing dependence.

Understanding this helps families anticipate future needs.

The Emotional Journey for Families

Each stage brings emotional challenges.

In the early stage:

- Uncertainty and denial

In the middle stage:

- Stress and frustration

In the late stage:

- Grief and emotional fatigue

Recognizing these emotions is important.

It helps families cope in a healthier way.

A Real-Life Reflection

A 70-year-old woman was diagnosed with early dementia.

Initially, she managed her daily activities with minimal support.

Over the next few years, she needed help with medications and household tasks.

Later, she required assistance with personal care.

In the final stage, she became fully dependent.

Her family, having understood the stages early, was better prepared.

They planned ahead, adjusted care, and focused on maintaining her dignity.

Myth vs Fact

Myth: Dementia progresses the same way in everyone.
Fact: While stages provide a general framework, progression varies widely from person to person.

Common Mistakes to Avoid

- Expecting the patient to function as before
- Delaying planning
- Ignoring safety concerns
- Not preparing emotionally

STAGES OF DEMENTIA

Dementia gets worse over time. Symptoms and daily challenges increase at each stage.

Stage	What Happens	Example
1. EARLY STAGE (Mild)	• Mild memory problems • Forgets recent events or names • May repeat questions • Independent in daily activities • Symptoms may be noticed by family and friends	Forgets where keys were placed but finds them later.
2. MODERATE STAGE (Moderate)	• Memory loss becomes worse • Trouble with planning and problem solving • Difficulty doing complex tasks • Needs help with some daily activities • Mood and behavior changes may occur	Forgets important dates or gets lost in familiar places.
3. MODERATELY SEVERE STAGE (Moderately Severe)	• Severe memory loss • Confusion about time and place • Trouble speaking and finding words • Needs help with most daily activities • Behavior changes increase	Forgets family members' names or needs help with dressing.
4. SEVERE STAGE (Severe)	• Very severe memory loss • Cannot communicate well • Needs help with all daily activities • May not recognize family or friends • More changes in behavior and personality	Cannot talk clearly or recognize loved ones.
5. VERY SEVERE STAGE (Very Severe / End Stage)	• Loss of ability to speak • Loss of movement and control • Needs full-time care • Trouble eating and swallowing • Increased risk of infections and complications	Bedridden, needs help with everything.

Every person is different. With care, support and understanding, quality of life can be improved at every stage.

Red Flag Warnings

- Rapid decline over a short period
- Frequent falls
- Difficulty swallowing
- Severe behavioral changes

Chapter Summary

Dementia progresses through early, middle, and late stages.
Each stage brings increasing cognitive and functional decline.
Understanding these stages helps families prepare and respond effectively.
Emotional support is essential throughout the journey.

Action Plan

- Learn the stages and what to expect
- Plan early for future needs
- Address safety concerns proactively
- Provide emotional support
- Focus on dignity at every stage

Transition to Next Chapter

Now that we understand how dementia progresses over time, the next step is to recognize the complications that can arise, so that families can act early to prevent or manage them effectively.

CHAPTER 11: Complications of Dementia – What Families Must Be Ready For

When Dementia Begins to Affect the Whole Body

In the earlier chapters, we focused on memory, thinking, and behavior.

But as dementia progresses, it becomes clear that this condition is not limited to the mind alone.

The brain controls almost every function in the body.

So when the brain is affected, the impact spreads.

Movement slows. Appetite changes. Balance becomes uncertain. Judgment weakens.

Gradually, complications begin to appear.

These complications are often not sudden. They develop quietly, over time.

Recognizing them early can prevent serious consequences.

Why Complications Develop

As dementia advances, the brain loses its ability to:

- Process information accurately
- Recognize needs such as hunger, thirst, or pain
- Coordinate movement
- Respond appropriately to the environment

A patient may not realize:

- They are thirsty
- They are in pain
- They are at risk of falling

This is not neglect.

It is the disease.

Understanding this helps families respond with awareness instead of frustration.

Falls and Injuries – A Major Turning Point

Falls are one of the most serious complications in dementia.

They occur due to:

- Poor balance
- Muscle weakness
- Confusion
- Unsafe surroundings

- Medication side effects

A fall can lead to:

- Fractures
- Hospitalization
- Sudden loss of independence

Very often, families notice a significant decline after a fall.

Doctor's Pearl

Preventing a fall is far more important than treating one. A single fall can change the course of the illness.

Malnutrition and Weight Loss

As dementia progresses, eating becomes more difficult.

Patients may:

- Forget to eat
- Lose interest in food
- Have difficulty using utensils
- Develop swallowing problems

This can lead to:

- Weight loss

- Weakness
- Increased risk of infections

Regular monitoring of nutrition becomes essential.

Infections – Often Subtle but Serious

Patients with dementia are more vulnerable to infections.

Common infections include:

- Urinary tract infections
- Pneumonia

In older adults, infections may not present with typical symptoms.

Instead, the first sign may be:

- Sudden confusion
- Increased agitation
- Reduced alertness

Early recognition is critical.

Medication Errors – A Preventable Risk

Managing medications becomes difficult over time.

Patients may:

- Forget doses
- Take extra doses
- Mix up medications

This can lead to serious complications.

Simple systems and supervision can prevent many of these errors.

Behavioral Complications

Behavioral changes can be distressing.

These may include:

- Agitation
- Aggression
- Wandering
- Suspicion
- Sleep disturbances

These behaviors are not intentional.

They are caused by changes in brain function.

Understanding this helps caregivers respond calmly.

Loss of Independence

Over time, patients lose the ability to perform daily tasks.

This includes:

- Dressing
- Bathing
- Cooking
- Managing finances

This loss is gradual but significant.

It requires increasing support.

Hospitalization – A High-Risk Situation

Hospital stays can be particularly challenging.

Reasons include:

- Unfamiliar environment
- Disruption of routine
- Increased risk of delirium

Even a short hospitalization can lead to noticeable decline.

Preventing avoidable hospitalizations is important.

Complications of Dementia

As dementia progresses, it can lead to several complications that affect health, safety and quality of life.

1 Falls and Injuries

Poor judgement, balance problems and weakness increase the risk of falls, fractures and head injuries.

2 Infections

Weak immune system and difficulty swallowing can lead to pneumonia, urinary tract infections and other infections.

3 Malnutrition and Dehydration

Memory problems, poor appetite and difficulty eating or drinking can cause weight loss and dehydration.

4 Difficulty Swallowing (Dysphagia)

Problems with swallowing can cause choking, aspiration and pneumonia.

5 Behavioral and Psychological Symptoms

Anxiety, agitation, depression, hallucinations and aggression can occur and be distressing for both the person and caregivers.

6 Loss of Independence

Difficulty with daily tasks leads to dependence on others for personal care, mobility and decision making.

7 Pressure Sores (Bedsores)

Long periods of sitting or lying down can cause sores on the skin, especially in the elderly.

8 Sleep Problems

Sleep disturbances, wandering at night and daytime sleepiness are common and lead to further health issues.

9 Wandering and Getting Lost

Disorientation can cause wandering, getting lost and may lead to serious injury or danger.

10 Emotional Stress for Caregivers

Caregivers may face stress, burnout, anxiety and depression while managing dementia care.

Early care, regular medical checkups, a safe environment and strong support can help prevent or reduce these complications.

Care, Support and Safety Make a Big Difference

A Real-Life Reflection

An 80-year-old man with moderate dementia had a fall at home.

He sustained a fracture and required hospitalization.

During his hospital stay, he became more confused and less mobile.

Before the fall, he was walking independently.

Afterward, he required assistance for most activities.

This is a common and important pattern.

Myth vs Fact

Myth: Dementia only affects memory.
Fact: Dementia affects physical health, safety, nutrition, and overall functioning.

Common Mistakes to Avoid

- Ignoring early signs of complications
- Delaying treatment for infections
- Assuming behavioral changes are intentional
- Neglecting fall prevention

Red Flag Warnings

- Sudden change in behavior or alertness
- Frequent falls
- Rapid weight loss
- Difficulty swallowing
- Signs of infection

Chapter Summary

Dementia affects multiple aspects of health beyond memory.
Falls, infections, malnutrition, and medication errors are common complications.
Behavioral changes and loss of independence are significant challenges.
Early recognition and prevention improve outcomes.

Action Plan

- Make the home environment safe
- Monitor nutrition and weight regularly
- Watch for early signs of infection
- Supervise medications
- Seek medical attention for sudden changes
- Maintain a structured daily routine

Transition to Next Chapter

Now that we understand the complications that can arise, the next step is to focus on lifestyle and non-medical strategies that can help maintain function and improve quality of life.

CHAPTER 12: Lifestyle and Non-Medical Care – The Daily Habits That Truly Help

Where Everyday Actions Make the Biggest Difference

When families first hear the diagnosis of dementia, their attention naturally turns to medications.

That is understandable.

But over many years of practice, I have seen something equally important.

What you do every day often matters just as much as what you prescribe.

Simple routines, a calm environment, regular movement, meaningful interaction, and good sleep can quietly shape the patient's daily experience.

These are not small measures.

They are powerful tools.

Why Daily Care Matters So Much

The brain affected by dementia struggles with change and complexity.

When life becomes unpredictable, confusion increases.

When life becomes structured and familiar, the mind feels more secure.

Routine reduces anxiety.
Familiarity builds comfort.

This is why daily habits are central to care.

Building a Simple and Predictable Routine

A steady routine is one of the most effective ways to reduce confusion.

Try to keep:

- Regular waking and sleeping times
- Fixed meal schedules
- Consistent bathing and personal care times
- Planned daily activities

When the day follows a pattern, the patient feels more settled.

Resistance to care often decreases.

Doctor's Pearl

Routine is not restriction. It is support. It gives the brain a sense of stability.

Physical Activity – Keep the Body Moving

Regular movement benefits both body and brain.

It helps:

- Improve balance and reduce falls
- Enhance mood
- Promote better sleep
- Maintain overall health

Activities do not need to be complex.

Simple options include:

- Walking
- Light stretching
- Chair exercises
- Guided gentle movements

Even 20 to 30 minutes a day can make a meaningful difference.

Consistency matters more than intensity.

Mental Engagement – Keeping the Mind Active

The brain benefits from gentle stimulation.

Helpful activities include:

- Reading simple material
- Looking at family photographs
- Listening to familiar music
- Playing simple games or puzzles
- Talking about past experiences

The key is to match the activity to the person's ability.

Too difficult can lead to frustration.
Too simple may not engage.

Balance is important.

Nutrition – Supporting Strength and Energy

Eating habits often change in dementia.

Patients may:

- Forget to eat
- Lose interest in food
- Have difficulty using utensils

Helpful strategies include:

- Offering small, frequent meals
- Providing familiar and simple foods
- Using easy-to-handle portions
- Encouraging regular fluid intake

Monitoring weight and hydration is essential.

Sleep – Restoring the Brain

Sleep disturbances are common.

Patients may:

- Have difficulty falling asleep
- Wake frequently at night
- Sleep during the day

Improving sleep can significantly improve behavior and function.

Helpful habits include:

- Keeping a regular sleep schedule
- Limiting daytime naps
- Reducing caffeine intake
- Creating a calm, quiet sleeping environment
- Ensuring exposure to natural daylight

Non-Medical Care in Dementia

Care, Support and Daily Strategies Improve Quality of Life

1. A Safe Environment

- Remove clutter and tripping hazards
- Good lighting
- Use labels and signs
- Lock dangerous areas

2. Daily Routine

- Keep a regular schedule
- Plan meals, activities and sleep time
- Predictable routine reduces anxiety

3. Communication

- Speak slowly and clearly
- Use simple words and short sentences
- Maintain eye contact
- Listen with patience

4. Nutrition

- Balanced, healthy meals
- Small, frequent meals
- Encourage fluids
- Make mealtime calm and pleasant

5. Physical Activity

- Regular light exercise like walking
- Improves mood and sleep
- Keeps the body active and strong

6. Mental Stimulation

- Engage in activities like reading, music, puzzles, crafts
- Encourages thinking and memory
- Keeps the mind active

7. Emotional Support

- Offer love, warmth and reassurance
- Avoid criticism or arguments
- Praise small achievements

8. Sleep Hygiene

- Maintain regular sleep time
- Avoid caffeine late in the day
- Keep the room quiet, dark and comfortable

Additional Helpful Strategies

- Involve in simple household tasks
- Encourage social interaction
- Allow time – do not rush
- Use reminders (notes, alarms, calendars)
- Provide choices, not commands
- Ensure personal dignity and respect

Caregiver Support

Caring for a person with dementia can be demanding. **Caregivers should also take care of their own health, seek support and take breaks.**

Kindness, patience and daily support make a big difference in the life of a person with dementia.

Support. Understand. Respect. Together we can make life better.

Social Interaction – A Powerful Influence

Human connection plays a vital role.

Isolation can worsen both mood and cognition.

Encourage:

- Conversations with family
- Time with friends
- Participation in small social activities
- Community or day programs

Even brief interactions can improve mood.

Creating a Supportive Environment

The home environment should be:

- Safe
- Simple
- Familiar

Helpful adjustments include:

- Good lighting
- Removing clutter
- Keeping frequently used items in the same place
- Using labels when needed

A calm environment reduces confusion and stress.

Managing Stress and Emotions

Patients may feel anxious or confused but may not express it clearly.

Caregivers can help by:

- Speaking calmly
- Using simple language
- Avoiding arguments
- Offering reassurance

Tone often matters more than words.

A Real-Life Reflection

A 74-year-old man with moderate dementia became restless and irritable in the evenings.

His family introduced a structured routine:

- Morning walk
- Quiet afternoon activity
- Early dinner
- Calm evening environment

Within weeks, his agitation reduced significantly.

No additional medication was needed.

Simple changes made a meaningful difference.

Myth vs Fact

Myth: Only medications can help dementia.
Fact: Daily routine, environment, and lifestyle play a major role in improving quality of life.

Common Mistakes to Avoid

- Keeping an irregular routine
- Expecting too much from the patient
- Ignoring sleep problems
- Allowing social isolation

Red Flag Warnings

- Significant weight loss
- Severe sleep disturbance
- Increasing agitation
- Frequent falls

Chapter Summary

Daily habits play a powerful role in dementia care.
Routine, physical activity, nutrition, sleep, and social interaction are essential.
A supportive environment reduces confusion and stress.
Simple, consistent measures can improve quality of life.

Action Plan

- Establish a consistent daily routine
- Encourage regular physical activity
- Provide appropriate mental stimulation
- Monitor nutrition and hydration
- Improve sleep habits
- Maintain social interaction
- Create a safe and calm home environment

Transition to Next Chapter

Now that we understand the importance of lifestyle and daily care, the next step is to explore medications used in dementia, what they can realistically achieve, and how to use them wisely.

CHAPTER 13: Medicines Used in Dementia Care – What They Can and Cannot Do

The Question Every Family Asks

Soon after the diagnosis is made, almost every family asks:

"Is there a medicine that will cure this?"

It is a natural question.

In most illnesses, we expect a treatment that brings things back to normal.

Dementia does not follow that pattern.

At present, there is **no medicine that can cure most types of dementia**.

But there are medications that can help.

Used appropriately, they may:

- Improve certain symptoms
- Slow decline in some patients
- Help maintain daily function for a period of time

Understanding their role clearly helps families use them wisely.

The Real Goal of Treatment

The purpose of medication in dementia is not reversal.

It is support.

Medications aim to:

- Improve communication between brain cells
- Stabilize symptoms for some time
- Support daily functioning
- Help manage mood and behavior when needed

These benefits are often modest, but they can be meaningful.

Two Main Groups of Medicines

Most commonly used medications fall into two groups:

1. Cholinesterase inhibitors
2. Memantine

Each works differently, but both aim to support brain function.

Cholinesterase Inhibitors – Supporting Brain Signals

These include medications such as donepezil, rivastigmine, and galantamine.

They work by increasing levels of acetylcholine, a chemical involved in memory and learning.

They are typically used in:

- Mild to moderate dementia
- Sometimes in later stages

Possible benefits:

- Slight improvement in memory and attention
- Temporary stabilization of symptoms

Limitations:

- Effects are usually modest
- They do not stop disease progression

Common side effects:

- Nausea
- Loss of appetite
- Diarrhea
- Sleep disturbance

Doctors usually start with a low dose and increase gradually.

Memantine – Regulating Brain Activity

memantine works through a different mechanism.

It regulates glutamate, a chemical involved in learning. Excess glutamate may contribute to brain cell damage.

Memantine is often used in:

- Moderate to severe dementia
- Sometimes in combination with other medications

Possible benefits:

- Modest improvement in thinking and function
- May help with behavior in some patients

Side effects are generally mild:

- Dizziness
- Headache
- Occasional confusion

Medicines for Mood, Sleep, and Behavior

Dementia often brings emotional and behavioral symptoms.

Medications may be used carefully for:

- Depression
- Anxiety
- Sleep disturbance
- Agitation or aggression

These may include antidepressants or selected sleep aids.

However, caution is essential.

Some medications, especially sedatives and certain antipsychotics, may increase:

- Risk of falls
- Confusion
- Stroke risk in older adults

They should be used only when clearly necessary and under supervision.

Medicines That Can Make Things Worse

Some medications can worsen cognitive function.

These include:

- Strong sedatives
- Certain antihistamines
- Some bladder medications
- Older anticholinergic drugs

Regular medication review is essential.

Doctor's Pearl

In dementia care, more medication is not always better. Careful and selective use is often safer and more effective.

What Families Should Expect

This is the most important point.

Medications may:

- Provide mild improvement
- Slow decline in some cases
- Help maintain independence for a period

They do not:

- Cure dementia
- Restore normal memory
- Stop progression completely

Setting realistic expectations helps families focus on overall care.

MEDICINES FOR DEMENTIA

Medicines can help manage symptoms, improve quality of life and support daily function. They do not cure dementia.

1. MEDICINES THAT MAY HELP MEMORY AND THINKING

MEDICINE CLASS	EXAMPLES	HOW THEY WORK	POTENTIAL BENEFITS
Cholinesterase Inhibitors	• Donepezil (Aricept®) • Rivastigmine (Exelon®) • Galantamine (Razadyne®)	Increase levels of a chemical (acetylcholine) in the brain that helps memory and thinking.	• May improve memory, attention and thinking • May slow down worsening of symptoms for some time • May help with daily activities
NMDA Receptor Antagonist	• Memantine (Namenda®)	Regulates glutamate, another brain chemical involved in learning and memory.	• May slow down worsening of symptoms • May help with behavior, communication and daily function

2. MEDICINES FOR BEHAVIORAL AND PSYCHOLOGICAL SYMPTOMS

MEDICINE CLASS	EXAMPLES	USED FOR	POTENTIAL BENEFITS
Antidepressants (SSRI)	• Sertraline (Zoloft®) • Citalopram (Celexa®) • Escitalopram (Lexapro®)	Depression, anxiety, irritability	Improve mood, reduce anxiety and agitation
Antipsychotics (Use with caution)	• Risperidone (Risperdal®) • Quetiapine (Seroquel®) • Olanzapine (Zyprexa®)	Severe agitation, aggression, hallucinations, delusions	May reduce severe symptoms Not for routine use – higher risk of side effects
Mood Stabilizers / Others	• Valproate (Depakote®) • Carbamazepine (Tegretol®) • Trazodone (Desyrel®)	Mood swings, agitation, sleep problems	May help control mood and improve sleep

3. MEDICINES ARE MOST EFFECTIVE WHEN

- ✔ Started in early to moderate stages
- ✔ Used regularly as prescribed
- ✔ Combined with non-medical care and support
- ✔ Monitored by a healthcare professional

4. COMMON SIDE EFFECTS

- Nausea, vomiting, diarrhea
- Loss of appetite, weight loss
- Dizziness, drowsiness
- Muscle cramps
- Confusion, worsening behavior (rare)

Report any side effects to your doctor.

5. IMPORTANT INFORMATION

- Take medicines as prescribed at the same time every day.
- Regular follow-up is important to check benefits and side effects.
- Do not stop medicines suddenly.
- Keep a list of all medicines and share with your doctor.
- Caregiver support is important for safe use of medicines.
- Contact your doctor if symptoms worsen or new problems occur.

Medicines are one part of care. Patience, understanding, structure and support make the biggest difference.

Always consult your doctor for the right treatment plan for your loved one.

A Real-Life Reflection

A 75-year-old woman with early dementia was started on donepezil.

Over the next year, her symptoms remained stable. She was able to continue her daily activities with some support.

Later, memantine was added as her condition progressed.

While decline continued gradually, the medications helped maintain her independence for a longer period.

This is a realistic outcome.

Myth vs Fact

Myth: Dementia medications can cure memory loss.
Fact: These medications may help symptoms and slow decline, but they do not cure the disease.

Common Mistakes to Avoid

- Expecting dramatic improvement
- Stopping medication too early
- Using multiple drugs without clear benefit
- Ignoring side effects

Red Flag Warnings

- Persistent nausea or loss of appetite
- Sudden increase in confusion after starting medication
- Excessive sleepiness or falls
- New behavioral changes

Chapter Summary

Medications play a supportive role in dementia care.
Cholinesterase inhibitors and memantine are the main treatments.
Benefits are modest but meaningful.
Careful use and monitoring are essential.
Realistic expectations improve outcomes.

Action Plan

- Discuss medication options clearly with your doctor
- Start medications gradually
- Monitor for benefits and side effects
- Review all medications regularly
- Focus on overall care, not just medication

Transition to Next Chapter

While current medications provide support, new and emerging treatments are offering additional hope. In the next chapter, we will explore these newer therapies and what they may mean for the future of dementia care.

CHAPTER 14: New and Emerging Treatments – Hope, Progress, and Practical Reality

A Changing Direction in Dementia Care

For many years, dementia treatment focused mainly on managing symptoms.

Families often felt that once the diagnosis was made, there was little that could change the course of the illness.

That view is beginning to shift.

Recent advances in research have introduced treatments that aim to act on the disease process itself, not just the symptoms.

This has brought hope.

At the same time, it is important to understand these developments clearly, without unrealistic expectations.

From Symptom Control to Disease Modification

Traditional medications help brain cells communicate better.

Newer therapies attempt something different.

They aim to:

- Target abnormal proteins in the brain
- Slow the underlying disease process
- Delay progression

In Alzheimer-type dementia, the focus has been on reducing amyloid accumulation in the brain.

This represents an important change in approach.

Monoclonal Antibody Therapies

Medications such as lecanemab and donanemab belong to this newer class.

They work by:

- Binding to amyloid protein
- Helping remove it from the brain

This is a significant scientific development.

However, it is essential to understand their role carefully.

Who May Benefit from These Treatments

These therapies are not suitable for all patients.

They are generally considered for:

- Early-stage Alzheimer-type dementia
- Mild cognitive impairment due to Alzheimer's disease
- Patients with confirmed amyloid presence

They are not typically used in advanced stages.

Careful patient selection is critical.

What Benefits Can Be Expected

Clinical studies suggest these treatments may:

- Slow the rate of cognitive decline
- Delay progression to more advanced stages

However:

- The benefit is modest
- Improvement is not dramatic
- Memory does not return to normal

This must be clearly understood before starting treatment.

Risks and Monitoring

These treatments require careful monitoring.

One important concern is **ARIA (Amyloid-Related Imaging Abnormalities)**.

This may include:

- Brain swelling
- Small areas of bleeding

Because of this, patients require:

- Screening before treatment
- Regular MRI scans
- Close follow-up

Certain individuals may be at higher risk and require special caution.

Doctor's Pearl

New treatments bring hope, but they are not simple or risk-free. Careful selection and monitoring are essential.

Practical Considerations

These therapies are not simple daily medications.

They often involve:

- Intravenous infusions
- Regular clinic visits
- Ongoing monitoring

Other factors include:

- Cost
- Availability
- Insurance coverage
- Patient suitability

Families must weigh the benefits against these practical considerations.

Other Areas of Ongoing Research

Research in dementia continues to evolve.

Current areas of investigation include:

- Therapies targeting tau protein
- Anti-inflammatory approaches
- Neuroprotective treatments
- Combination therapies

While promising, many of these are still under study.

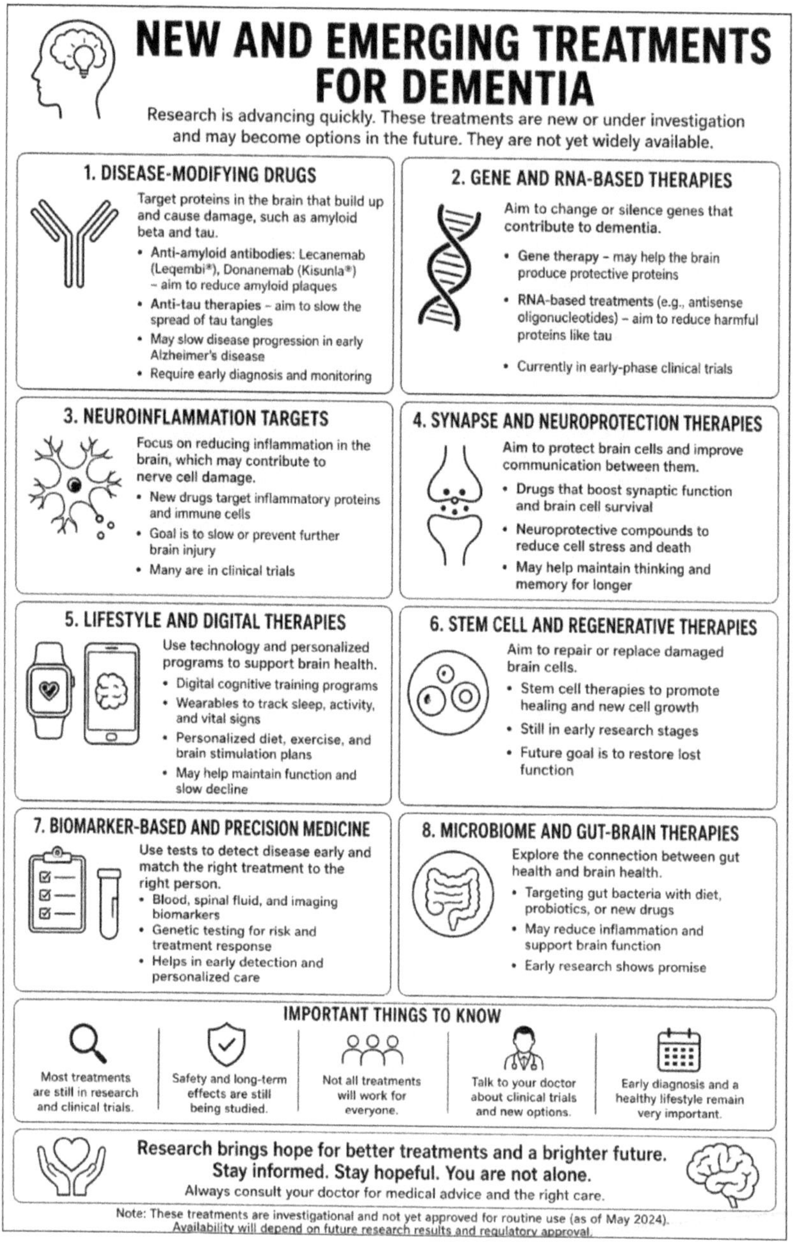
NEW AND EMERGING TREATMENTS FOR DEMENTIA
Research is advancing quickly. These treatments are new or under investigation and may become options in the future. They are not yet widely available.
1. DISEASE-MODIFYING DRUGS
Target proteins in the brain that build up and cause damage, such as amyloid beta and tau.
• Anti-amyloid antibodies: Lecanemab (Leqembi®), Donanemab (Kisunla®) – aim to reduce amyloid plaques
• Anti-tau therapies – aim to slow the spread of tau tangles
• May slow disease progression in early Alzheimer's disease
• Require early diagnosis and monitoring
2. GENE AND RNA-BASED THERAPIES
Aim to change or silence genes that contribute to dementia.
• Gene therapy – may help the brain produce protective proteins
• RNA-based treatments (e.g., antisense oligonucleotides) – aim to reduce harmful proteins like tau
• Currently in early-phase clinical trials
3. NEUROINFLAMMATION TARGETS
Focus on reducing inflammation in the brain, which may contribute to nerve cell damage.
• New drugs target inflammatory proteins and immune cells
• Goal is to slow or prevent further brain injury
• Many are in clinical trials
4. SYNAPSE AND NEUROPROTECTION THERAPIES
Aim to protect brain cells and improve communication between them.
• Drugs that boost synaptic function and brain cell survival
• Neuroprotective compounds to reduce cell stress and death
• May help maintain thinking and memory for longer
5. LIFESTYLE AND DIGITAL THERAPIES
Use technology and personalized programs to support brain health.
• Digital cognitive training programs
• Wearables to track sleep, activity, and vital signs
• Personalized diet, exercise, and brain stimulation plans
• May help maintain function and slow decline
6. STEM CELL AND REGENERATIVE THERAPIES
Aim to repair or replace damaged brain cells.
• Stem cell therapies to promote healing and new cell growth
• Still in early research stages
• Future goal is to restore lost function
7. BIOMARKER-BASED AND PRECISION MEDICINE
Use tests to detect disease early and match the right treatment to the right person.
• Blood, spinal fluid, and imaging biomarkers
• Genetic testing for risk and treatment response
• Helps in early detection and personalized care
8. MICROBIOME AND GUT-BRAIN THERAPIES
Explore the connection between gut health and brain health.
• Targeting gut bacteria with diet, probiotics, or new drugs
• May reduce inflammation and support brain function
• Early research shows promise
IMPORTANT THINGS TO KNOW
Most treatments are still in research and clinical trials.
Safety and long-term effects are still being studied.
Not all treatments will work for everyone.
Talk to your doctor about clinical trials and new options.
Early diagnosis and a healthy lifestyle remain very important.
Research brings hope for better treatments and a brighter future.
Stay informed. Stay hopeful. You are not alone.
Always consult your doctor for medical advice and the right care.
Note: These treatments are investigational and not yet approved for routine use (as of May 2024).
Availability will depend on future research results and regulatory approval.

A Real-Life Reflection

A 65-year-old patient with early Alzheimer-type dementia was evaluated for newer treatment.

After detailed discussion about benefits and risks, the patient and family chose to proceed.

Over time, the decline appeared slower than expected.

However, regular follow-up and imaging were required.

The family felt the decision was worthwhile, but they understood the limitations.

This balanced approach is important.

Myth vs Fact

Myth: New dementia treatments can cure the disease.
Fact: Current therapies may slow progression in selected patients, but they do not cure dementia.

Common Mistakes to Avoid

- Assuming these treatments are suitable for everyone
- Expecting rapid or dramatic improvement
- Ignoring potential risks
- Starting treatment without proper evaluation

Red Flag Warnings

- New neurological symptoms after starting treatment
- Severe headache or confusion
- Changes in balance or coordination
- Sudden worsening of condition

Chapter Summary

New treatments are changing the approach to dementia care.
Monoclonal antibodies target the disease process in Alzheimer-type dementia.
Benefits are modest and mainly seen in early stages.
Careful patient selection and monitoring are essential.
Hope must be balanced with realistic expectations.

Action Plan

- Discuss eligibility for new treatments with your doctor
- Understand benefits and risks clearly
- Confirm diagnosis before starting therapy
- Commit to regular monitoring if treatment is chosen
- Make informed and balanced decisions

Transition to Next Chapter

While medical treatments continue to evolve, one of the most immediate challenges families face is managing behavioral and emotional changes. In the next chapter, we will focus on understanding these behaviors and responding with patience and compassion.

CHAPTER 15: Managing Difficult Behaviors – Responding with Patience, Not Panic

When Behavior Becomes the Hardest Part

For many families, the most difficult part of dementia is not memory loss.

It is behavior.

A calm person may become irritable.
A cooperative parent may resist care.
A gentle spouse may become suspicious or withdrawn.

These changes can be painful and confusing.

They can also feel very personal.

But there is one important truth to hold on to:

These behaviors are not intentional.

They are the result of changes in the brain.

When we understand this, our response changes.

Why Behavioral Changes Occur

Dementia affects parts of the brain responsible for:

- Judgment
- Emotional control
- Perception
- Communication

The patient may feel:

- Confused
- Anxious
- Frightened

But may not be able to express it clearly.

Behavior becomes a form of communication.

Instead of asking, "Why is this happening?"
It is often more helpful to ask, "What might be causing this?"

Agitation and Aggression

Agitation may appear as:

- Restlessness
- Pacing
- Irritability

Aggression may include:

- Shouting
- Resistance to care

- Physical agitation

Common triggers include:

- Pain or discomfort
- Fatigue
- Noise or overstimulation
- Change in routine
- Feeling rushed

How to respond:

- Stay calm
- Speak gently
- Avoid arguing
- Give space when needed
- Identify and address possible triggers

Doctor's Pearl

Do not take difficult behavior personally. The disease is speaking, not the person.

Wandering and Getting Lost

Wandering is common and can be dangerous.

Patients may:

- Walk aimlessly

- Try to leave home
- Search for something or someone

Possible reasons include:

- Restlessness
- Confusion
- Need for activity

Helpful strategies:

- Maintain a consistent routine
- Provide safe walking opportunities
- Use supervision when needed
- Ensure identification is available

Suspicion and Paranoia

Patients may develop false beliefs.

They may feel:

- Someone is stealing from them
- They are being harmed
- Familiar people are strangers

These beliefs feel real to them.

How to respond:

- Do not argue
- Offer calm reassurance
- Redirect attention

- Check for underlying causes

Hallucinations

Some patients may see or hear things that are not present.

This is more common in certain types of dementia.

Approach:

- Stay calm
- Do not dismiss their experience harshly
- Reassure gently
- Ensure safety
- Seek medical advice if needed

Sleep Problems and Evening Confusion

Many patients become more confused or restless in the evening.

This is often referred to as "sundowning."

Sleep-related issues may include:

- Difficulty falling asleep
- Frequent waking
- Daytime sleepiness

Helpful steps:

- Maintain regular sleep timing
- Encourage daytime activity
- Limit long daytime naps
- Create a calm evening environment

Resistance to Care

Patients may resist:

- Bathing
- Dressing
- Taking medications

This can be frustrating.

Better approaches:

- Do not rush
- Break tasks into simple steps
- Offer choices
- Try again later if needed

Communication Makes a Difference

How we speak has a strong impact.

Helpful techniques:

- Use short, simple sentences
- Speak slowly
- Maintain eye contact
- Avoid complex instructions
- Use reassurance rather than correction

Tone often matters more than words.

A Real-Life Reflection

A 76-year-old woman became very agitated during bathing.

Her family initially tried to complete the task quickly, which made her more resistant.

They changed their approach:

- Explained calmly before starting
- Slowed down the process
- Allowed her to participate
- Stopped when she became distressed

Over time, her agitation reduced significantly.

Small changes in approach made a large difference.

MANAGING DIFFICULT BEHAVIOUR IN DEMENTIA

Behaviours are a way of communicating unmet needs.
Patience, understanding and the right approach can help.

1. COMMON DIFFICULT BEHAVIOURS

Agitation	Aggression	Wandering	Apathy	Hallucinations & Delusions	Repetition
Restless, anxious or unable to relax	Hitting, pushing, shouting or threatening	Walking aimlessly, getting lost or leaving home	Lack of interest, no motivation, not participating	Seeing or hearing things that are not real	Asking the same questions or repeating actions

2. KEY STRATEGIES TO MANAGE DIFFICULT BEHAVIOUR

Identify the Cause
Look for triggers such as pain, hunger, tiredness or changes in routine.

Communicate Calmly
Use a calm tone, simple words and short sentences.

Create a Calm Environment
Reduce noise and clutter. Ensure good lighting and comfortable surroundings.

Establish Routine
Keep a regular daily routine for meals, activities and sleep.

Provide Reassurance
Offer comfort and let them know they are safe and cared for.

Validate Feelings
Acknowledge their feelings. This reduces stress and anxiety.

Ensure Safety
Remove hazards and ensure a safe environment.

Seek Support
Ask for help from family, friends or professionals.

3. WHAT TO AVOID

- Arguing or correcting
- Raising your voice
- Rushing or crowding
- Taking it personally
- Sudden changes

4. WHEN TO SEEK HELP

- Behaviour is severe or frequent
- Risk of harm to self or others
- Sudden change in behaviour
- Suspected pain or illness

5. MEDICAL TREATMENTS

If strategies don't work, a doctor may consider medicines for specific symptoms.

Always consult your doctor.

6. CAREGIVER SELF-CARE

- Take breaks and rest
- Talk about your feelings
- Manage stress and relax
- Look after your health
- Accept help when offered

**Kindness, patience and consistency make a big difference.
You are making a difference every day.**

★ You are not alone. Help and support are always available.

Myth vs Fact

Myth: Behavioral problems are due to stubbornness.
Fact: These behaviors are caused by brain changes and are not under the patient's control.

Common Mistakes to Avoid

- Arguing with the patient
- Taking behavior personally
- Rushing care activities
- Ignoring triggers

Red Flag Warnings

- Sudden severe agitation
- New hallucinations
- Behavior that risks safety
- Rapid behavioral changes

Chapter Summary

Behavioral changes are common in dementia.
They are caused by changes in the brain, not intention.
Understanding triggers helps manage these behaviors.
Calm communication and patience are essential.

Action Plan

- Identify possible triggers for behavior
- Maintain a calm and consistent routine
- Use simple and gentle communication
- Avoid arguments
- Ensure safety at all times
- Seek medical advice when needed

Transition to Next Chapter

Managing behavior is essential, but ensuring safety in daily life is equally important. In the next chapter, we will focus on practical steps to make the home environment safer while preserving independence as much as possible.

CHAPTER 16: Safety at Home, Driving, and Everyday Decisions – Protecting Without Taking Away Dignity

When Safety Quietly Becomes the Priority

In the early stages of dementia, safety concerns are occasional.

A missed dose of medication.
A stove left on once.
A door not locked properly.

Families notice these events, correct them, and move on.

But as the condition progresses, these are no longer isolated incidents.

They become patterns.

And at that point, safety is no longer a small issue. It becomes central to daily care.

The real challenge is not only to keep the patient safe.

It is to do so without making them feel controlled, restricted, or diminished.

That balance requires thought, patience, and sensitivity.

Why Safety Risks Increase

Dementia affects the brain's ability to:

- Recognize danger
- Make sound decisions
- Follow steps
- Remember instructions

A patient may not understand that something is unsafe.

They may forget instructions given just minutes earlier.

They may misjudge situations that were once simple.

This is not carelessness.

It is the disease.

Understanding this helps caregivers respond with patience rather than frustration.

Falls – A Common and Serious Risk

Falls are one of the most important safety concerns.

They occur due to:

- Poor balance

- Muscle weakness
- Confusion
- Cluttered surroundings
- Medication side effects

A fall can lead to:

- Fractures
- Hospitalization
- Sudden decline in function

Very often, patients do not fully recover their previous level of independence after a major fall.

Doctor's Pearl

Preventing a fall is one of the most effective ways to preserve independence in dementia care.

Making the Home Safer

Small changes can make a significant difference.

Consider:

- Removing loose rugs and clutter
- Improving lighting, especially at night
- Installing grab bars in bathrooms
- Using non-slip mats
- Keeping frequently used items within easy reach

The goal is not to change the home completely.

It is to simplify it.

Kitchen Safety – A Hidden Risk

Cooking can become unsafe.

Patients may:

- Forget to turn off the stove
- Leave food unattended
- Use appliances incorrectly

Helpful strategies include:

- Supervising cooking
- Simplifying meal preparation
- Using appliances with automatic shut-off
- Limiting access when necessary

At some point, independent cooking may no longer be safe.

Medication Safety – Preventing Mistakes

Medication errors are common and potentially dangerous.

Patients may:

- Forget doses
- Take extra doses
- Confuse different medications

Helpful solutions:

- Pill organizers
- Pre-filled medication boxes
- Clear labeling
- Caregiver supervision

Keeping the system simple is essential.

Driving – A Difficult but Necessary Conversation

Driving represents independence.

Giving it up is emotionally challenging.

However, dementia affects:

- Reaction time
- Judgment
- Navigation
- Decision-making

Warning signs include:

- Getting lost

- Missing traffic signals
- Slow reaction
- Near accidents

Approach the conversation early.

When possible:

- Involve the patient
- Be respectful and calm
- Offer alternatives such as family support or transportation services

Safety must always come first.

Wandering – Planning Ahead

Wandering can be dangerous.

Patients may leave home unexpectedly and be unable to return.

Preventive steps include:

- Maintaining a regular routine
- Supervising when needed
- Using simple monitoring systems
- Ensuring identification is available

Preparation is essential.

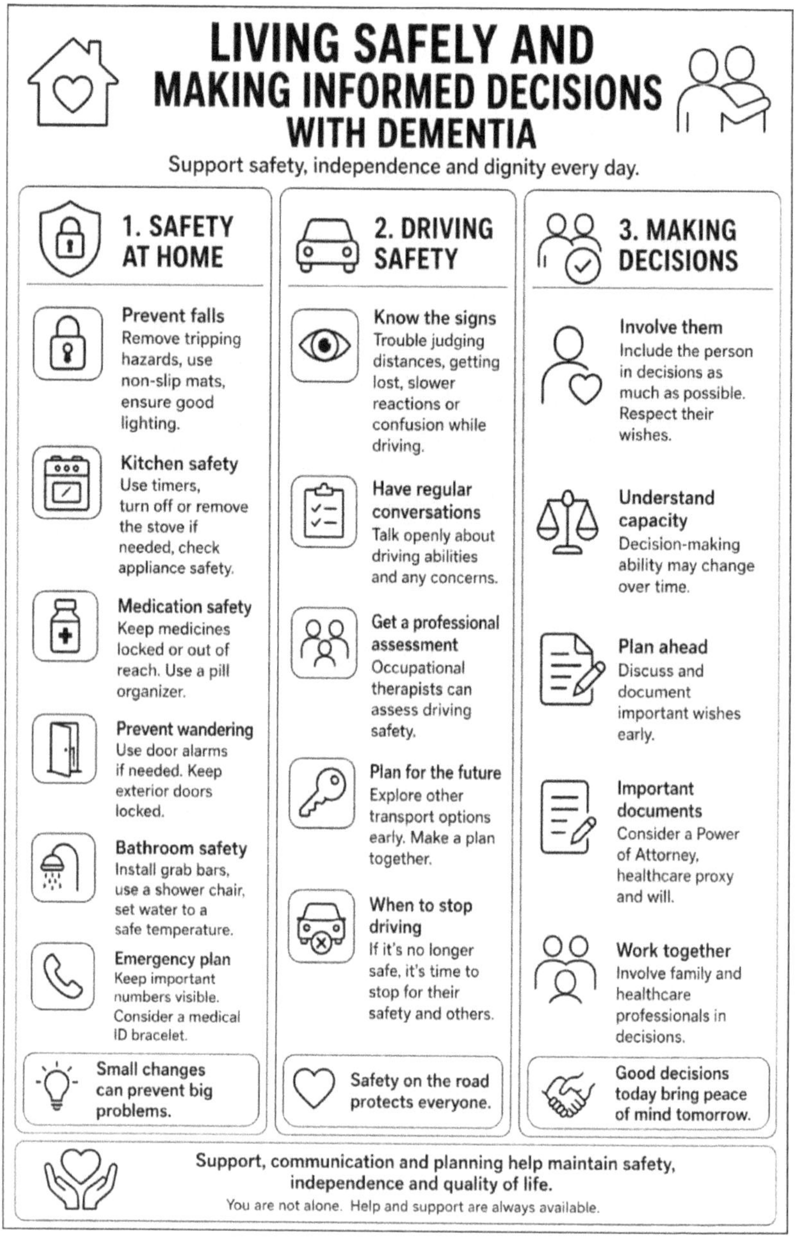
LIVING SAFELY AND
MAKING INFORMED DECISIONS
WITH DEMENTIA
Support safety, independence and dignity every day.
1. SAFETY AT HOME
Prevent falls
Remove tripping hazards, use non-slip mats, ensure good lighting.
Kitchen safety
Use timers, turn off or remove the stove if needed, check appliance safety.
Medication safety
Keep medicines locked or out of reach. Use a pill organizer.
Prevent wandering
Use door alarms if needed. Keep exterior doors locked.
Bathroom safety
Install grab bars, use a shower chair, set water to a safe temperature.
Emergency plan
Keep important numbers visible. Consider a medical ID bracelet.
Small changes can prevent big problems.
2. DRIVING SAFETY
Know the signs
Trouble judging distances, getting lost, slower reactions or confusion while driving.
Have regular conversations
Talk openly about driving abilities and any concerns.
Get a professional assessment
Occupational therapists can assess driving safety.
Plan for the future
Explore other transport options early. Make a plan together.
When to stop driving
If it's no longer safe, it's time to stop for their safety and others.
Safety on the road protects everyone.
3. MAKING DECISIONS
Involve them
Include the person in decisions as much as possible. Respect their wishes.
Understand capacity
Decision-making ability may change over time.
Plan ahead
Discuss and document important wishes early.
Important documents
Consider a Power of Attorney, healthcare proxy and will.
Work together
Involve family and healthcare professionals in decisions.
Good decisions today bring peace of mind tomorrow.
Support, communication and planning help maintain safety, independence and quality of life.
You are not alone. Help and support are always available.

Financial Safety – Protecting Against Mistakes

Dementia affects financial judgment.

Patients may:

- Make unusual purchases
- Fall for scams
- Give away money

Helpful measures:

- Monitoring accounts
- Simplifying finances
- Setting alerts
- Limiting access when necessary

Early action prevents serious consequences.

Balancing Safety and Independence

This is one of the most delicate parts of caregiving.

Too little supervision increases risk.

Too much control can lead to frustration and loss of dignity.

The goal is to:

- Support independence where possible
- Intervene when necessary
- Adjust gradually as the condition progresses

There is no perfect formula.

But thoughtful balance makes a difference.

A Real-Life Reflection

A 73-year-old man with moderate dementia began leaving the stove on and forgetting to lock doors.

His family introduced simple changes:

- Installed stove safety devices
- Added door alerts
- Organized medications
- Created a structured routine

These steps improved safety without making him feel restricted.

This is the goal.

Myth vs Fact

Myth: Safety measures take away independence.
Fact: Thoughtful safety measures protect independence by preventing injuries and crises.

Common Mistakes to Avoid

- Ignoring early safety concerns
- Making sudden, drastic changes
- Not involving the patient in decisions
- Delaying necessary restrictions

Red Flag Warnings

- Repeated unsafe behavior
- Getting lost
- Medication errors
- Financial confusion

Chapter Summary

Safety becomes increasingly important as dementia progresses.
Falls, medication errors, driving, and wandering are major concerns.
Simple home modifications can reduce risk.
Balancing safety and dignity is essential.

Action Plan

- Assess the home for safety hazards
- Simplify cooking and medication routines
- Address driving concerns early
- Take steps to prevent wandering
- Protect financial resources
- Maintain a safe and supportive environment

Transition to Next Chapter

As safety needs increase, so does the responsibility on caregivers. In the next chapter, we will focus on caregiver stress, emotional burden, and how to maintain your own well-being while caring for your loved one.

CHAPTER 17: The Hidden Impact of Dementia on Caregivers and Families – Stress, Love, Loss, and Strength

The Illness That Affects the Whole Family

When we talk about dementia, we often focus on the patient.

But in real life, dementia does not stay confined to one person.

It slowly enters the entire family.

It changes routines.
It reshapes relationships.
It tests patience and emotional strength in ways few other conditions do.

Behind every patient, there is a caregiver.

And behind that caregiver, there is often a family trying to adjust, cope, and keep life moving forward.

This chapter is about that side of the story.

How Caregiving Begins – Almost Without Notice

Caregiving rarely starts with a clear decision.

It begins quietly.

A reminder about a medication.
Help with an appointment.
A little extra supervision.

At this stage, it feels manageable.

But over time, the demands grow.

More involvement.
More responsibility.
More emotional strain.

What began as occasional help becomes a daily commitment.

And often, caregivers do not realize how much their life has changed until they begin to feel overwhelmed.

The Emotional Burden – Complex and Often Unspoken

Caregivers experience a wide range of emotions.

They may feel:

- Love and commitment
- Frustration and impatience
- Guilt for feeling frustrated
- Sadness and grief

Among these, guilt is one of the most common.

"I should be more patient."
"I should not feel irritated."

These thoughts are very common.

It is important to understand:

These emotions are not a sign of failure.

They are a human response to a difficult situation.

Doctor's Pearl

Feeling tired, frustrated, or overwhelmed does not make you a bad caregiver. It means you are carrying a heavy responsibility.

Changing Relationships – A Quiet Form of Loss

Dementia changes relationships in a deep and gradual way.

A spouse may lose the companionship they once shared.

Conversations become shorter. Decisions become one-sided.

Over time, the relationship shifts from partnership to caregiving.

This creates a unique kind of grief.

Not sudden, but slow.

This is often described as **anticipatory grief**.

You are mourning the gradual loss of the person as you knew them.

Impact on Spouses

For spouses, the impact is often the most intense.

They may experience:

- Emotional loneliness
- Increased responsibility
- Physical exhaustion
- Social withdrawal

The person they depended on is now depending on them.

This role reversal can be emotionally painful.

THE IMPACT OF DEMENTIA ON CAREGIVERS

Caring for a loved one with dementia is loving and meaningful, but it can also be challenging.

1. COMMON IMPACTS ON CAREGIVERS

Emotional Stress
Worry, sadness, guilt and feeling overwhelmed.

Physical Tiredness
Fatigue, poor sleep and health problems.

Financial Strain
Extra costs and possible reduced income.

Social Isolation
Less time for friends, hobbies and activities.

Time Demands
Caregiving can be time-consuming and never really ends.

2. TIPS FOR CAREGIVER WELL-BEING

Take Care of Yourself
Your health matters. Eat well, rest and stay active.

Seek Support
Talk to family, friends or support groups. You are not alone.

Take Breaks
Respite care and short breaks can help you recharge.

Plan and Organize
Make lists, set priorities and ask for help.

Manage Stress
Try deep breathing, meditation, prayer or activities you enjoy.

Accept Your Feelings
It's okay to feel many emotions. Be kind to yourself.

3. USE AVAILABLE RESOURCES

Respite Services
Temporary care gives you time to rest and take care of other needs.

Support Groups
Share experiences and learn from others who understand.

Counseling
Professional support can help you cope and feel better.

Education
Learn about dementia and care strategies to feel more confident.

Community Resources
Local programs can provide help and services.

4. WHEN TO SEEK HELP

Seek help from a healthcare professional if you experience:

- Constant sadness or anxiety
- Trouble sleeping or relaxing
- Feeling hopeless or overwhelmed
- Thoughts of harming yourself

You deserve support. Reaching out shows strength.

Caregivers make a big difference every day. Take care of yourself so you can continue to care for your loved one.

You are not alone. Help and support are always available.

Impact on Children and Family Members

Adult children face a different kind of pressure.

They often need to:

- Balance caregiving with work and their own family
- Make important decisions for their parent
- Manage financial and legal responsibilities

Younger family members may feel confused or anxious.

They may not fully understand what is happening.

Open and simple communication helps reduce fear.

The Physical Toll on Caregivers

Caregiving affects the body as well as the mind.

Caregivers often:

- Sleep less
- Eat irregularly
- Skip their own medical care

Over time, this leads to:

- Fatigue
- Reduced immunity
- Increased risk of illness

Taking care of your own health is essential, not optional.

Caregiver Burnout – When the System Is Overloaded

Burnout develops slowly.

It may show as:

- Constant exhaustion
- Irritability
- Feeling overwhelmed
- Loss of interest in daily life
- Depression or anxiety

Many caregivers ignore these signs.

They feel they must continue no matter what.

But ignoring burnout can lead to serious physical and emotional consequences.

Doctor's Pearl

You cannot provide good care if you are completely exhausted. Taking care of yourself is part of caregiving.

Financial and Career Impact

Dementia care can affect financial stability.

Caregivers may:

- Reduce working hours
- Take time off
- Spend more on healthcare and support services

This can create long-term financial stress.

Planning ahead helps reduce this burden.

Social Isolation – A Hidden Challenge

Many caregivers gradually withdraw from social life.

Reasons include:

- Lack of time
- Fatigue
- Difficulty leaving the patient alone

This leads to isolation.

Isolation increases stress and emotional burden.

Maintaining some level of connection is important.

Support Systems – You Do Not Have to Do This Alone

Caregiving should not be a one-person effort.

Support can come from:

- Family members
- Friends
- Community resources
- Support groups
- Professional caregivers

Asking for help is not weakness.

It is a necessary step.

Respite Care – Taking a Break Without Guilt

Respite care provides temporary relief.

Options include:

- Help from family
- Professional home care
- Adult day care programs
- Short-term facility care

Even short breaks can restore energy and perspective.

They improve both caregiver health and patient care.

Finding Meaning in the Journey

Despite the challenges, many caregivers find something unexpected.

A sense of meaning.

They may discover:

- Emotional strength
- Deep commitment
- A renewed sense of purpose

Some families grow closer.

Some relationships deepen in new ways.

This does not remove the hardship, but it adds value to the journey.

A Real-Life Reflection

A 65-year-old woman caring for her husband once said:

“This is not the life we planned. But I know I am doing what matters.”

That quiet strength reflects the reality of caregiving.

Myth vs Fact

Myth: A good caregiver should handle everything alone.
Fact: Dementia care requires support. Seeking help is a sign of strength.

Common Mistakes to Avoid

- Trying to manage everything alone
- Ignoring personal health
- Feeling guilty for normal emotions
- Avoiding support systems

Red Flag Warnings

- Severe exhaustion
- Depression or anxiety
- Anger toward the patient
- Neglect of personal health

Chapter Summary

Dementia affects the entire family.
Caregivers face emotional, physical, and financial challenges.

Burnout is common and should be recognized early.
Support and respite care are essential.
Caregiving, though difficult, can also bring meaning and strength.

Action Plan

- Recognize your limits
- Ask for help and share responsibilities
- Take regular breaks
- Maintain your own health
- Stay socially connected
- Seek support groups or counseling
- Accept your emotions without guilt

Transition to Next Chapter

As caregiving continues, it becomes important to plan ahead for legal, financial, and long-term decisions. In the next chapter, we will focus on how to prepare for the future with clarity and confidence.

CHAPTER 18: Legal, Financial, and Long-Term Planning – Making Wise Decisions Early

The Conversations Most Families Delay

In my experience, this is one of the most important parts of dementia care.

And often, it is the most delayed.

Families hesitate.

They feel uncomfortable.
They worry about upsetting the patient.
They hope things will remain stable for a long time.

But dementia is a progressive condition.

Over time, the ability to make decisions declines.

If planning is delayed too long, families may be forced to make urgent decisions without clear guidance.

That is when stress, confusion, and even conflict can arise.

Planning early is not about fear.

It is about respect, clarity, and protection.

Involving the Patient Early – A Gift to the Future

In the early stage, the patient can still:

- Understand information
- Express preferences
- Participate in decisions

This is the best time to talk.

Important areas to discuss include:

- Medical care preferences
- Living arrangements
- Financial decisions
- Future caregiving plans

These conversations should be:

- Calm
- Respectful
- Honest

When patients are involved early, they feel heard and respected.

And families gain clarity for the future.

Doctor's Pearl

Decisions made early, while the patient can still participate, prevent confusion and conflict later.

Advance Directives – Honoring Medical Wishes

Advance directives are legal documents that record a person's wishes about medical care.

They may include:

- Preferences about life-sustaining treatment
- Decisions regarding hospitalization
- End-of-life care choices

These documents guide doctors and families when the patient can no longer communicate clearly.

They reduce uncertainty and help ensure that care aligns with the patient's values.

Power of Attorney – Choosing the Right Person

As dementia progresses, someone must make decisions on behalf of the patient.

Two important roles are:

Medical Power of Attorney

- Makes healthcare decisions

Financial Power of Attorney

- Manages finances, bills, and assets

Choosing the right person is critical.

This should be someone who is:

- Trustworthy
- Responsible
- Able to act in the patient's best interest

Wills and Estate Planning

A will ensures that assets are distributed according to the patient's wishes.

Without a will, the process becomes more complicated and may not reflect what the patient intended.

Early planning allows:

- Clear decisions
- Reduced family conflict
- Smoother transition of assets

Understanding the Cost of Care

Dementia care can become expensive, especially in later stages.

Costs may include:

- Medications
- Home care services
- Adult day care
- Assisted living
- Nursing facility care

Planning ahead helps families prepare financially and avoid unexpected stress.

Medicare and Medicaid – A Basic Understanding

Many families are uncertain about coverage.

Medicare

- Covers medical services
- Limited coverage for long-term care

Medicaid

- May cover long-term care for eligible individuals
- Based on financial criteria

Understanding these programs early helps in planning.

In more complex situations, professional advice may be helpful.

Protecting Against Financial Mistakes and Scams

Dementia affects judgment.

Patients may:

- Make unusual purchases
- Give away money
- Fall victim to scams

Protective steps include:

- Monitoring accounts
- Setting alerts
- Simplifying finances
- Limiting access when necessary

Early action can prevent serious financial loss.

Planning for Long-Term Care

At some point, families must decide where care will be provided.

Options include:

- Home care with support
- Assisted living
- Memory care units
- Nursing facilities

Each option has advantages and challenges.

Planning early allows time to:

- Explore choices
- Visit facilities
- Make thoughtful decisions

A Real-Life Reflection

A 67-year-old man with early dementia worked with his family to complete advance directives and assign power of attorney.

He clearly expressed his wishes.

Years later, when his condition progressed, his family made decisions with confidence.

There was no confusion or conflict.

Planning early made a significant difference.

Myth vs Fact

Myth: Legal and financial planning can wait until later.
Fact: Delaying planning often leads to confusion, conflict, and loss of control.

Common Mistakes to Avoid

- Avoiding difficult conversations
- Delaying legal documentation
- Choosing the wrong decision-maker
- Ignoring financial planning

Red Flag Warnings

- Unpaid bills
- Unusual spending
- Financial confusion
- Family disagreements

Chapter Summary

Early planning is essential in dementia care.
Advance directives and power of attorney protect patient wishes.
Understanding costs helps families prepare.
Planning reduces stress and prevents complications.

Action Plan

- Discuss future care preferences early
- Complete advance directives
- Assign medical and financial power of attorney
- Update wills
- Understand healthcare coverage
- Monitor and protect financial resources
- Begin planning for long-term care

Transition to Next Chapter

As dementia progresses further, care needs become more complex and sensitive. In the next chapter, we will focus on advanced dementia and how to provide care with dignity, comfort, and compassion.

CHAPTER 19: Advanced Dementia – Care with Dignity, Comfort, and Compassion

When the Goal of Care Gently Shifts

As dementia moves into its later stages, something important changes.

In the earlier stages, our focus is on maintaining independence, slowing decline, and managing symptoms.

In advanced dementia, the focus becomes different.

Now, the priority is **comfort, dignity, and quality of life**.

This is not giving up.

It is a thoughtful and compassionate shift in care.

When families understand this transition, decisions become clearer and more peaceful.

What Advanced Dementia Looks Like

In advanced dementia, the changes are significant.

Patients may:

- Lose the ability to communicate clearly
- No longer recognize familiar faces
- Become unable to walk independently
- Have difficulty swallowing
- Depend completely on others for daily care

Daily life becomes simple.

Eating, comfort, positioning, and gentle interaction become the main concerns.

Even in this stage, the patient continues to experience:

- Comfort and discomfort
- Calm and distress

Care should always focus on these experiences.

Communication Without Words

When speech becomes limited, communication does not stop.

Patients may express themselves through:

- Facial expressions
- Eye movements
- Body language
- Sounds or gestures

A calm tone, a gentle touch, and a familiar presence can be deeply reassuring.

At this stage, how we say something matters more than what we say.

Doctor's Pearl

Even when memory and language fade, the ability to feel comfort and kindness remains. Gentle care always matters.

Eating and Swallowing – A Sensitive Challenge

Swallowing problems are common in advanced dementia.

Patients may:

- Take longer to swallow
- Cough during meals
- Refuse food
- Lose weight

This increases the risk of choking and infections.

Helpful approaches include:

- Offering soft or modified foods
- Feeding slowly and patiently

- Keeping the patient upright during meals

Decisions about feeding support should be made carefully, with respect for the patient's wishes and overall condition.

Infections and Medical Decisions

Infections become more frequent in advanced stages.

Common examples:

- Pneumonia
- Urinary tract infections

Families may face difficult decisions:

- Hospital care versus home care
- Aggressive treatment versus comfort-focused care

These decisions should be guided by:

- The patient's earlier wishes
- Overall quality of life
- Medical advice

There is no single correct answer.

Each situation is personal.

ADVANCED DEMENTIA CARE

Focus on comfort, dignity and quality of life.
You are not alone. Support is available.

1. WHAT TO EXPECT

Progressive Changes
More help needed with daily care, communication, eating and mobility.

Increased Dependency
Rely on others for most or all activities.

Communication Changes
Words may be limited. Comfort and presence matter most.

Eating Challenges
Swallowing may be difficult. Risk of weight loss and illness.

Focus on Comfort
Goal is comfort, not cure. Every moment matters.

2. KEY AREAS OF CARE

Comfort First	Manage pain, breathlessness, constipation and other discomforts. Keep them clean, dry and comfortable.
Emotional Connection	Your voice, touch and presence bring comfort. Use simple words, gentle tone and reassurance.
Personal Care	Gentle hygiene, regular position changes and skin care help prevent discomfort and pressure sores.
Nutrition and Hydration	Offer favorite foods and small amounts often. Follow safe swallowing guidelines.
Safety	Prevent falls, infections and choking. Ensure a calm, safe environment.
Dignity and Respect	Involve them as much as possible. Respect their life story, values and preferences.

3. DECISIONS AND PLANNING

- Plan ahead: Advance care plan, Power of Attorney, healthcare proxy.
- Discuss wishes for medical care, resuscitation and end-of-life care.
- Review and update plans regularly.

4. END-OF-LIFE CARE

- Focus on comfort, not prolonging life.
- Hospice and palliative care can provide expert support.
- Keep loved ones close and meaningful moments matter.

5. CAREGIVER SUPPORT

Accept Help
Let others help with care and daily tasks.

Take Breaks
Rest and time for yourself prevent burnout.

Seek Support
Talk to family, friends or support groups. You are not alone.

Look After Your Health
Eat well, stay active and manage stress.

Know Where to Find Help
Reach out to doctors, hospice or local resources.

You are doing an incredible job.
Compassion, patience and love make all the difference.

Palliative Care – Focusing on Comfort

Palliative care focuses on:

- Relief of pain and discomfort
- Management of symptoms
- Improving quality of life

It can be introduced at any stage, but becomes especially important in advanced dementia.

The goal is not to cure.

The goal is to comfort.

Hospice Care – Support in the Final Phase

Hospice care is considered when the disease is advanced and life expectancy is limited.

It provides:

- Medical care
- Emotional support
- Guidance for families

Hospice can be provided at home or in a care facility.

It helps ensure that the final phase is peaceful and dignified.

Supporting the Family

This stage is emotionally very difficult.

Families may experience:

- Grief
- Emotional fatigue
- Uncertainty

Support is essential.

Talking openly, seeking help, and accepting emotions are important steps.

No one should go through this stage alone.

Maintaining Dignity at All Times

Dignity must remain central.

This includes:

- Respecting the patient's wishes
- Maintaining cleanliness and comfort
- Speaking respectfully
- Avoiding unnecessary interventions

Even in the final stage, dignity matters deeply.

A Real-Life Reflection

An 82-year-old woman with advanced dementia became unable to communicate and eat independently.

Her family chose comfort-focused care at home.

With hospice support, her symptoms were managed gently.

She remained comfortable, and her family spent meaningful, peaceful time with her.

This approach brought a sense of closure and calm.

Myth vs Fact

Myth: Nothing can be done in advanced dementia.
Fact: Comfort, dignity, and quality of life can always be improved.

Common Mistakes to Avoid

- Focusing only on aggressive treatment
- Ignoring the patient's wishes
- Delaying palliative or hospice care

- Neglecting emotional support

Red Flag Warnings

- Difficulty swallowing
- Frequent infections
- Severe weight loss
- Loss of mobility
- Increasing distress

Chapter Summary

Advanced dementia requires a shift toward comfort-focused care.
Communication continues even without words.
Feeding and infections become central concerns.
Palliative and hospice care provide essential support.
Dignity must be maintained at all times.

Action Plan

- Focus on comfort and quality of life
- Use gentle communication
- Manage feeding carefully
- Discuss care goals with healthcare providers
- Consider palliative and hospice care
- Support family members emotionally

Transition to Next Chapter

As families move through this stage, many questions naturally arise. In the next chapter, we will address common questions and provide clear, practical answers to guide you further.

CHAPTER 20: Frequently Asked Questions – Clear, Honest Answers When You Need Them Most

When Questions Keep Coming Back

Even after understanding dementia, questions remain.

They do not come in order.
They come during daily life.
They come when something unexpected happens.

Sometimes they are practical.
Sometimes they are emotional.

Families often hesitate to ask, thinking they should already know the answer.

But in dementia care, asking questions is not a weakness.

It is a sign of thoughtful caregiving.

In this chapter, I have answered the questions I hear most often in real practice, in a simple and direct way.

Is Dementia the Same as Alzheimer's Disease

No.

Alzheimer's disease is the most common cause of dementia, but it is not the only one.

There are several other types, including vascular dementia, Lewy body dementia, and frontotemporal dementia.

Understanding the type helps guide expectations and care.

Is Memory Loss Always Dementia

No.

Memory problems can occur due to:

- Normal aging
- Depression
- Medication side effects
- Sleep problems
- Vitamin deficiencies

This is why proper evaluation is essential.

Not every memory problem is dementia.

Can Dementia Be Cured

At present, most types of dementia cannot be cured.

However:

- Some causes of memory problems are reversible
- Treatments can help symptoms
- Newer therapies may slow progression in selected cases

The focus is on improving quality of life.

How Fast Does Dementia Progress

There is no single answer.

Progression varies from person to person.

Some decline slowly over many years.
Others progress more quickly.

Factors that influence progression include:

- Type of dementia
- Overall health
- Presence of other medical conditions
- Level of care and support

When Should Driving Stop

Driving should be reconsidered when:

- The person gets lost
- Reaction time slows
- Judgment becomes impaired
- Near accidents occur

This is often a difficult discussion.

It is better to address it early and plan alternatives.

Can Dementia Be Prevented

Not completely.

But risk can be reduced.

Helpful measures include:

- Controlling blood pressure, diabetes, and cholesterol
- Staying physically active
- Eating a healthy diet
- Maintaining good sleep
- Staying mentally and socially engaged

These steps support brain health.

Should the Patient Be Told About the Diagnosis

In most cases, yes.

Patients have the right to know, especially in the early stage.

The conversation should be:

- Honest
- Gentle
- Supportive

Each situation is different and should be handled thoughtfully.

How Do I Handle Repeated Questions

This is very common.

Instead of becoming frustrated:

- Answer calmly
- Keep responses simple
- Redirect attention when possible

Repetition is due to memory loss, not intention.

What Should I Do If the Patient Becomes Aggressive

Stay calm.

Then:

- Look for possible triggers such as pain or discomfort
- Avoid confrontation
- Give space
- Speak gently

Seek medical advice if behavior becomes severe.

When Is It Time for Additional Help or Facility Care

Consider additional help when:

- Safety becomes difficult
- Caregiver stress increases
- Medical needs become complex
- Daily care requires constant support

Seeking help is a responsible decision.

How Do I Take Care of Myself as a Caregiver

This is essential.

Caregivers should:

- Take regular breaks
- Seek support
- Maintain their own health
- Accept help from others

You cannot provide good care if you are exhausted.

Is It Normal to Feel Overwhelmed

Yes.

Feelings such as:

- Frustration
- Sadness
- Fatigue

are very common.

Acknowledging these emotions is important.

Support makes a difference.

What Matters Most in Dementia Care

At the end of the day, the most important elements are simple.

- Patience
- Kindness
- Respect
- Consistency

Even when memory fades, these still matter deeply.

Doctor's Pearl

Clear understanding reduces fear. When families know what to expect, they respond with confidence.

Common Mistakes to Avoid

- Avoiding questions due to fear
- Relying on unreliable information
- Ignoring caregiver needs
- Delaying important decisions

Red Flag Warnings

- Sudden worsening of symptoms
- Unsafe behavior
- Severe caregiver stress
- Lack of support

Chapter Summary

Dementia raises many questions for patients and families.
Clear answers reduce confusion and anxiety.
Every situation is unique and requires thoughtful decisions.
Understanding leads to better care.

Action Plan

- Ask questions openly
- Seek reliable information
- Discuss concerns with family
- Plan ahead
- Take care of your own well-being

Transition to Next Chapter

As we come to the final chapter of this book, we will bring together everything we have learned and focus on moving forward with clarity, compassion, and confidence.

CHAPTER 21: Conclusion – Moving Forward with Clarity, Compassion, and Strength

A Journey That Changes Everything

If you have reached this final chapter, you have already taken an important step.

You have moved from uncertainty toward understanding.

Dementia is not an easy condition to face. It affects memory, thinking, independence, and relationships. It changes daily life in ways that can feel overwhelming at times.

But there is another truth that is equally important.

With the right understanding, this journey becomes clearer.
With the right approach, it becomes more manageable.

You may not control the disease, but you can shape how you respond to it.

And that makes a meaningful difference.

What We Have Learned Together

Throughout this book, we have walked through dementia step by step.

We have understood:

- How memory changes begin
- What dementia truly means
- Early warning signs and Mild Cognitive Impairment
- Different types and causes
- Reversible conditions that must not be missed
- Risk factors and ways to protect brain health
- How diagnosis is made
- Newer tests and emerging treatments
- The stages of progression
- Complications and daily challenges
- Lifestyle care and medications
- Behavioral changes and safety
- Caregiver stress and support
- Legal, financial, and long-term planning
- Advanced care and end-of-life decisions

Each of these pieces is important.

Together, they form a complete and practical guide.

Clarity Reduces Fear

One of the greatest difficulties in dementia is uncertainty.

Not knowing what is happening.
Not knowing what will come next.

When we understand the condition, fear begins to reduce.

Clarity allows better decisions.
Better decisions lead to better care.

Even in difficult situations, understanding provides direction.

Compassion Is the Heart of Care

Medical knowledge is essential.

But in dementia care, compassion is just as important.

The person living with dementia is not just a patient.

They are someone who has lived a full life. Someone who has loved, worked, and built relationships.

Even when memory fades, the need for:

- Respect
- Kindness
- Reassurance

remains.

Simple actions matter.

A calm voice.
A gentle touch.
A patient response.

These often matter more than complex interventions.

For Caregivers – A Personal Message

If you are caring for someone with dementia, I want to speak to you directly.

What you are doing is not easy.

It requires patience, strength, and emotional resilience.

There will be difficult days.

Days when you feel tired.
Days when you feel frustrated.
Days when you feel uncertain.

These feelings are normal.

You are not alone.

Taking care of yourself is not optional.

It is necessary.

When you care for your own health, you are better able to care for your loved one.

Doctor's Pearl

In dementia care, perfection is not the goal. Consistent, compassionate care is what truly matters.

Holding On to What Still Matters

Dementia changes many things.

But it does not take away everything.

The ability to feel comfort remains.
The need for connection remains.

Even in advanced stages, these human elements continue.

Focusing on these brings meaning to the journey.

Looking Ahead with Strength

While we cannot control every aspect of dementia, we can control our response.

We can:

- Plan ahead
- Provide thoughtful care

- Create a safe environment
- Seek support when needed

Strength does not mean having all the answers.

It means continuing to move forward, step by step.

A Final Reflection

Dementia may take away certain abilities.

But it does not take away the value of a person.

Every stage of life deserves dignity.
Every patient deserves respect.
Every caregiver deserves support.

Chapter Summary

Dementia is a challenging but manageable condition.
Understanding reduces fear and improves decision-making.
Compassion is central to good care.
Caregivers need support and self-care.
Dignity and respect must be maintained at every stage.

Final Action Plan

- Continue learning and staying informed
- Plan early and revisit plans over time
- Provide care with patience and compassion
- Take care of your own health
- Seek help when needed
- Focus on dignity and quality of life

Closing Message

This journey is not easy.

But with knowledge, patience, and compassion, you can make a meaningful difference.

In the life of your loved one.

And in your own.

APPENDIX 1: A Simple Home Safety Checklist for Dementia Care

Why This Matters

A safe environment prevents injuries, reduces anxiety, and allows the patient to function with more confidence.

Small changes can make a big difference.

General Home Safety

- Keep pathways clear and free of clutter
- Remove loose rugs or secure them firmly
- Ensure good lighting in all rooms
- Install night lights in hallways and bathrooms
- Keep frequently used items within easy reach

Bathroom Safety

- Install grab bars near toilet and shower
- Use non-slip mats

- Keep water temperature moderate
- Ensure adequate lighting at night

Kitchen Safety

- Use appliances with automatic shut-off
- Supervise cooking when needed
- Keep sharp objects stored safely
- Avoid leaving the stove unattended
- Simplify meal preparation

Bedroom Safety

- Keep bed at a comfortable height
- Ensure easy access to bathroom
- Use night lights
- Avoid clutter near the bed

Fall Prevention

- Encourage proper footwear
- Avoid slippery floors
- Use walking aids if needed
- Review medications that may affect balance

Wandering Prevention

- Keep doors secure when needed
- Use simple monitoring systems
- Ensure patient carries identification
- Maintain a consistent routine

Medication Safety

- Use pill organizers
- Label medications clearly
- Keep a fixed medication schedule
- Supervise when necessary

Key Takeaway

Safety is not about restriction. It is about protection with dignity.

APPENDIX 2: Daily Care Plan Template for Caregivers

Why a Daily Plan Helps

A structured routine reduces confusion and improves cooperation.

Sample Daily Routine

Morning

- Wake up at the same time
- Personal hygiene and dressing
- Breakfast
- Light physical activity

Midday

- Lunch
- Rest or quiet activity
- Social interaction or simple engagement

Afternoon

- Light activity (walk, music, conversation)
- Snack and hydration

Evening

- Dinner at a fixed time
- Calm activity (TV, music)
- Prepare for sleep

Night

- Maintain a quiet, comfortable environment
- Keep lighting soft
- Ensure easy access to bathroom

Tips for Success

- Keep the routine simple
- Avoid sudden changes
- Be flexible when needed
- Focus on comfort, not perfection

Key Takeaway

A predictable day creates a calm mind.

APPENDIX 3: Caregiver Self-Care Plan

Why This Is Essential

Caregivers often neglect their own health.

This leads to burnout, which affects both caregiver and patient.

Daily Self-Care Checklist

- Eat regular, healthy meals
- Stay physically active, even briefly
- Take short breaks during the day
- Maintain your own medications and doctor visits

Emotional Health

- Talk to someone you trust
- Join a support group if possible
- Accept your emotions without guilt

Practical Support

- Share responsibilities with family
- Use respite care when needed
- Accept help without hesitation

Warning Signs of Burnout

- Constant fatigue
- Irritability
- Feeling overwhelmed
- Loss of interest in daily life

If these appear, take action early.

Key Takeaway

Taking care of yourself is part of taking care of your loved one.

APPENDIX 4: Questions to Ask Your Doctor

At the Time of Diagnosis

- What type of dementia is this
- What stage is the condition
- What tests are needed
- Are there reversible causes

About Treatment

- What medications are appropriate
- What benefits can be expected
- What are possible side effects
- Are new treatments an option

About Daily Care

- What lifestyle changes are helpful
- What safety precautions are needed
- When should driving stop

About Progression

- What changes should we expect
- When should we seek help
- What are warning signs

About Planning

- When should legal planning be done
- What long-term care options are available

Key Takeaway

Clear questions lead to clear care.

APPENDIX 5: 30-Day Action Plan for Families Facing Dementia

Week 1: Understanding and Evaluation

- Schedule medical evaluation if not done
- Review medications
- Begin observing symptoms carefully
- Start open family discussion

Week 2: Safety and Routine

- Assess home safety
- Create a simple daily routine
- Address immediate safety concerns
- Begin medication organization

Week 3: Health and Lifestyle

- Improve diet and hydration
- Start regular physical activity
- Address sleep issues

- Encourage mental engagement

Week 4: Planning and Support

- Begin legal and financial planning
- Identify support systems
- Explore community resources
- Plan follow-up care

Ongoing

- Monitor changes regularly
- Adjust care as needed
- Maintain caregiver health
- Focus on quality of life

Key Takeaway

Small steps taken early create long-term stability.

Thank You and Please Review the Book

Thank you for taking the time to read this book. I sincerely hope it has helped you understand your health a little more clearly and has given you practical, everyday steps you can follow with confidence. If you found this book helpful, **I would truly appreciate it if you could leave a brief and honest review.** Even a few lines sharing your experience can make a meaningful difference. Your feedback helps other readers find reliable, trustworthy health information and supports them in making better decisions for themselves and their families.

Warm regards,

Dr Prabhat Das

Continue your Healthcare Journey with these Books

Good health is a journey, not a single step. It is not achieved in one day or with one book. That is why I created the "Better Health with Dr Das Series", with each book addressing a different common condition. If you would like easy, practical guidance on other everyday health concerns, you may wish to explore the rest of books in this series.

Books in this series:

- Better Health starts Here: A Doctor's Guide to Staying Healthy After 40
- A Doctor's Easy Guide to Understanding & Managing OBESITY
- Doctor, What DIET Is Best for Me?
- Doctor, Why Can't I Lose Weight? A Doctor's Guide to Safe & Sustainable Weight Loss)
- A Doctor's Easy Guide to GLP-1 for Obesity
- A Doctor's Easy Guide to Understanding & Managing HIGH BLOOD PRESSURE
- A Doctor's Guide to Living Well With DIABETES
- A Doctor's Guide to Understanding & Managing THYROID DISEASES
- A Doctor's Guide to Understanding & Managing HIGH CHOLESTEROL
- A Doctor's Practical Guide to HEART HEALTH After 40: How to Protect Your Heart & Live Longer
- A Doctor's Guide to Healing & Reversing FATTY LIVER DISEASE: Simple, Natural & Science-Based Steps to Reduce Liver Fat and Prevent Complications

- Control Your ACID REFLUX, HEARTBURN & GERD: A Doctor's Practical Guide that Works
- Live Comfortably with IRRITABLE BOWEL SYNDROME: A Doctor's Practical Guide to Understanding & Managing IBS
- A Doctor's Practical Guide to Understanding & Managing GALLBLADDER STONES & OTHER PROBLEMS
- Take Control of COPD: A Doctor's Practical Guide to Better Breathing
- Living Better with ASTHMA: A Doctor's Practical Guide to Asthma Control
- SLEEP APNEA, INSOMNIA & OTHER SLEEP DISORDERS: A Doctor's Practical Guide to Better Sleep & Better Health
- Protect Your KIDNEYS: A Doctor's Practical Guide to Kidney Health & Prevention
- PROSTATE HEALTH: A Doctor's Practical Guide to Early Detection & Care
- ARTHRITIS: A Doctor's Practical Guide to Pain Control & Mobility
- STROKE: A Doctor's Practical Guide to Prevention & Early detection
- HEART ATTACK: A Doctor's Practical Guide to Prevention & Early detection
- CANCER: A Doctor's Practical Guide to Prevention & Early detection
- BACK PAIN: A Doctor's Practical Guide to Fixing Step by Step
- COMMON SKIN & HAIR PROBLEMS: A Doctor's Practical Guide to Skin & Hair Care
- DEMENTIA & MEMORY LOSS: A Doctor's Practical Guide to Prevention & Management
- Doctor, Why Am I TIRED All the Time? Fixing Fatigue & Getting Your Energy Back

www.ingramcontent.com/pod-product-compliance
Lightning Source LLC
LaVergne TN
LVHW020854300926
849194LV00002B/14
* 9 7 8 1 9 7 1 6 7 2 7 0 0 *